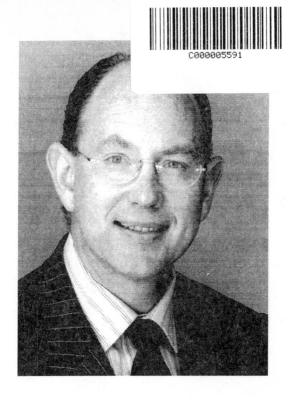

DAVID H.A. O'CONNELL was born in Cork, Ireland, in 1955. He was educated at Presentation Brothers College and studied medicine at University College, Cork. His postgraduate training was completed in London. He settled in Chelsea, where he has been in General Practice for the past fifteen years. In addition he has worked for some years as an aero-medical repatriation physician for International Assistance Services, flying around the world to bring home patients who have become seriously ill abroad. He acts as medical adviser to a number of companies and private organizations, for whom he has been advising on jetlag for some time. Outside of work his interests include wine and travel, literature and polo.

JETLAG
How To Beat It

Dr David H.A. O'Connell

MB BCh BAO DRCOG
MICGP FRSH FRIPHH

Foreword by Anthony Holden

Preface by Anne Robinson

ASCENDANT PUBLISHING

First published in 1997 by Ascendant Publishing
PO Box 16113, London SW3 3WA, Great Britain

© David H.A. O'Connell 1997
Foreword © Anthony Holden 1997
Preface © Anne Robinson 1997

Cover-page author photograph by Francis Loney
Smiles Studio, 2 Uxbridge Street, London W8 7SY

Typeset by Black Ace Editorial
PO Box 6557, Forfar, DD8 2YS, Scotland

Printed in England by Redwood Books
Kennet Way, Trowbridge, BA14 8RN

A CIP catalogue record for this book
is available from the British Library

ISBN   0–9531345–0–4

ACKNOWLEDGEMENTS

I am deeply indebted to the many authors and researchers whose scientific papers provide so much of the ground-work for this book, to the many captains, co-pilots, flight engineers and cabin staff who have answered so many questions for me, to the many patients who have taken the time to explain and discuss the problems they encounter with jetlag, and to the staff of the library of the Royal Society of Medicine and the British Library for helping me to track down some often obscure references.

Special thanks to Janette White for her help with the manuscript, and also to Black Ace for their editorial input.

*This book is dedicated to
the memory of E.O.C. and to B.M.*

*The former who taught me
the value of hard work,
and the latter who ensures
I do not forget.*

CONTENTS

FOREWORD

As a writer and journalist I was a frequent long-haul flier, for business as much as pleasure, even before I married an American wife – since when I have inevitably become a more frequent long-haul flier than ever. Like most regular travellers I know, I tried gamely to take jetlag in my own amateur stride, finding it worse going one way than the other (though never remembering which), and settling the whole pesky business with an improvized, often futile blend of sleeping pills and 'keeping going'.

As a result, I have managed to fall asleep at all the wrong times, making a chump of myself while conducting important interviews, even missing them altogether. Once, taking a post-lunch siesta in Los Angeles the day after arriving from London, I woke up to realize I had slept through the dinner for which I had been freshening up, missing the chance to sit next to Lauren Bacall.

As I advance further into middle age, I find the jetlag problem gets no better while the long-haul travel gets worse. As well as some half a dozen trips a year to the States, including my annual pilgrimages to the world championships of poker in Las Vegas and our family's summer holiday at Cape Cod, exciting chances to visit the Far East, Australasia and the South Pacific still come my way as a travel writer for the *Times*.

For years I have been seeking an authoritative guide

to dealing with jetlag, though I cannot really take all the credit for the fact that the man I consulted in the meantime – my doctor and friend, David O'Connell – was fast becoming a world authority on the subject.

Now, at last, David has blessed the world with all the information it needs, in a smart, slim volume the right size to fit in your hand baggage, alongside your timetable, there to be consulted whenever the need arises.

Like me, I'll bet, you sophisticated globetrotters never realized what you were up against when coping with those drooping eyelids, all those aches and pains. Well, now you know: circadian rhythms, zeitgeibers and hypoxia, not to mention barotrauma, hyperventilation and 25 hours in a day. Don't worry; ahead lie explanations of all this which even I can understand. Melatonin, whose potential benefits are clearly explained, is one possible solution of which we all wanted to learn more. Claret was another some of us had tried, without dreaming we might, in some circumstances, be doing the right thing. Light and shade, noise and silence, plus of course the optimum use of time itself, are all things we have long needed help with.

And now we've got it.

In his own inimitable way, familiar to those of us lucky enough to be his patients, Dr O'Connell spells out the scientific aspects of everyday matters in detail which will fascinate the reader not least because his own fascination shines through so clearly. Whether dealing with symptom or cure, the problems of cabin air pressure or when to lie down in a darkened hotel room, with a damp towel on your brow, 'Doc' David is now there to hold our hands, tut-tut if we do the wrong thing, and rescue us from ourselves.

For some, he will help maximize the use of travel time to the welcome advantage of their business lives.

For others, he will add a fun-filled day or two to a long-haul holiday. For all, he will banish jetlag where it belongs – back to the blue yonder, strictly for the birds.

Anthony Holden
London, July 1997

PREFACE

I have lost count of the hours I have spent in hotel rooms across America and in the Far East watching television as the dawn breaks. As well as the wasted afternoons when I should have been working or better still enjoying myself but instead was fast asleep. My body and my time clock unable for days to adjust to being eight hours behind in California. Or eight hours ahead in Hong Kong.

I do not exaggerate. Jetlag, in its time, has caused me to temporarily dip into the most dreadful depression and panic. So what a glorious relief to find a doctor taking jetlag seriously. It's given me permission to take it seriously too. And after a lifetime of accepting I will need half the holiday to recover from the flight. Or half of the next month to recover from the holiday. I now follow a simple procedure that sees me through the worst in the first twenty-four hours.

I can't believe my luck and good fortune. I am astonished, in fact, that no-one has seen fit to address this pressing problem before.

Perhaps one of the reasons is because male business executives are apt to put a macho gloss on their ability to cope with the effects of international travel. They boast of crossing time zones as if this were ordinary and natural and exhilarating and fun. What remains a secret is how often faulty calls and bad judgements are made while the same allegedly carefree executives are disorientated. Or how much better a meeting or negotiation might have been if he who was attending it was of sound mind. Instead of spaced out, fearful and weary.

For the first time I've learnt the particular effects on women of jetlag and see how important it is for those on HRT or the Pill to be aware of what is happening to their bodies when they travel large distances at great speed.

Not everybody will be able to adapt their schedules to make full use, every trip, of Dr O'Connell's well researched wisdom. You need decent airlines, no huge delays, appropriate destinations and co-operative colleagues in order to make the very most of this invaluable book. But I urge you to give it a go.

All you have to do is persuade yourself that jetlag is a very real medical condition that deserves treatment. Then all the strategy to deal with the problem is here. Most of it so deceptively simple that I'm furious I didn't work it out for myself.

It certainly works for me. I thank David O'Connell for extending our family holiday enjoyment and for improving the quality of my life on foreign working trips. He has released me from a lifetime's tyranny without me having to take a single pill. I hope he can do the same for you.

Anne Robinson
London, August 1997

IMPORTANT NOTE

What follows is the considered opinion and advice of the author, himself a highly qualified and experienced doctor, and having regard to the published medical evidence. Please note, however, that the advice contained herein is of necessity in general terms, and should only be followed in particular cases if endorsed by each reader's own personal physician. This requirement particularly applies to anyone suffering from any pre-existing medical condition or who is currently taking any form of medication. All applications of the advice, suggestions and treatments put forward in this book are at the reader's own discretion and responsibility.

To be as realistic as possible, the flight examples considered in this book are authentic and are believed to be correct at the time of going to press. They should not be relied upon, however, for the purpose of making travel arrangements. This is because airlines update their flight numbers and times on a regular basis; some every three months, others every six months. Even where flight numbers and times are changed, it is likely that their durations will remain similar. The examples presented in this book will thus retain their illustrative value. But for up-to-date factual accuracy, the reader should always consult a reliable travel agent or the airlines direct.

INTRODUCTION

This book has been written for you: the long-suffering long-distance traveller. Jetlag is the bane of twentieth-century travel. It has been responsible for countless failed business deals, ruined holidays and less-than-happy honeymoons.

Despite its often disastrous effects, jetlag, until now, has received surprisingly little sympathy from employers and hardly a mention in medical textbooks.

During the 1980s I had an increasing number of patients who complained of diverse conditions such as insomnia and other sleep disturbances, anxiety, depressive disorders, bowel upsets and general malaise. The one factor common to these patients was that they all, in the course of their work, undertook international travel on a regular basis.

The question therefore suggested itself: what common cause, or causes, gave rise to these widespread symptoms?

Meanwhile, as part of my own clinical work involved my travelling to the far corners of the world to repatriate patients who had become ill abroad, I noticed that I myself was suffering from some of the complaints that my patients were describing to me. Following a trip of several days to either the Far East or the Americas I would be afflicted by a malaise and a mental lethargy. I could function, but did not enjoy doing so. This condition could last for up to a week before spontaneous recovery ensued.

My searches of the available medical literature were at first disappointing. There were no medical textbooks on the subject of jetlag. There were no medical experts in this field who lectured to doctors or ran symposia to enable we clinicians to better understand this condition and convey the fruits of research to our patients in the form of meaningful and effective treatment.

I decided therefore to examine the subject piecemeal – starting with the basic sciences of physiology, anatomy and comparative biology, then working upwards through general medicine, endocrinology and pharmacology, and finally to aerospace and aviation medicine – to draw together the large but disparate body of information that was known about matters relating to jetlag. In the course of my studies I found that many of the most valuable research contributions have been made by colleagues working in aviation and aerospace medicine, i.e., where their 'guinea pigs' are pilots (usually fighter pilots) and astronauts, and where the demand for practical benefits is both understandable and intense.

Finally, after many months of study, and practical testing of my theories, I had a clearer understanding of what was happening to my patients, and correspondingly of how I could help them.

And help you too, perhaps?

Even if you belong to the happy minority who appear not to suffer from jetlag, this book should enable you to sympathize with, and allow for, the very real discomforts and maladies to which your less fortunate colleagues and employees are liable. And if you are a sufferer from jetlag, this book should at least equip you to minimize that suffering. It is offered as a simple distillation of current scientific understanding of the problems, and a programme of practical remedies for overcoming them.

I hope you find it useful.

David O'Connell
Chelsea, London
Summer 1997

1

The Normal Circadian Cycle

Jetlag is a highly unpleasant physical, psychological and emotional condition that arises when our inbuilt 24-hour clock is out of synchronization with the stimuli we are receiving from the outside world. In medical terms this is known as circadian rhythm desynchronosis.

Circadian comes from the Latin *circa* (about) and *dies* (a day).

In order to understand how the jetlag situation arises, it is first necessary to grasp what happens to us when we choose to stay put in the same place on earth, and live our lives day after day without ever travelling through time zones.

We all remember how, as children, we were sent to bed when it was getting dark and roused again from sleep by our parents once morning had come. Later we learned to repeat this pattern without prompting and even in our 'rebellious' college years we seldom strayed much outside this routine; because, when we did, we would find that if we stayed up all night partying or even just cramming for exams – went to bed at say 5 a.m. and got up at midday – we would feel very much the worse for wear.

It is only in adult life, when we have a career involving a great deal of international travel or shift work, that these physiological limitations (i.e., of confining activity to daytime, and sleeping by night) which we previously took for granted become a serious problem.

For practical purposes, most humans will be asleep for about eight hours between approximately midnight and 8 a.m., and will be awake and active for the remaining sixteen hours between 8 a.m. and midnight.

Most of us can also identify with one of two types:

The 'larks' are people who rise earlier than others in the morning. They can't sleep in. They feel most energetic in the mornings and are then at their most productive. After dinner their thoughts turn to bed and sleep.

The 'owls' do not enjoy getting up in the morning and will stay in bed as long as possible. They take a long time to get going. They do not become really productive until the afternoon. After dinner they really get into their stride and usually stay up after everyone else has gone to bed. An owl will then happily work away on some project until the small hours of the morning – burning the midnight oil.[1,2]

As people age they are less likely to remain owls and are prone to adopt more larklike habits.[3]

At this stage you should take note of which category you fall into and try to preserve this daily architecture both at home and abroad. For example, Winston Churchill would often work until 3–4 a.m. each night and spend the mornings in bed with his dispatch boxes, quite often giving dictation notes to his secretary through the bathroom door while having his morning bath, thus making him an owl.[4]

Sir Colin Marshall of British Airways is said to be up and at his desk very early each day, which would make him a lark.[5]

Lady Thatcher was reputed to start her day very early but also work through to very late each night, making her a combination of owl and lark during her premiership.[6]

During these two different periods vastly different processes are taking place in the body:

Respiration, or breathing rate, slows down during the night.[7] The metabolic rate in the body is much lower during sleep.[8] The body temperature is much higher during wakefulness than sleep.[9] There is a decrease in heart rate and blood pressure during sleep[10] and a rise in electrical skin resistance.[11] Activity in the gastrointestinal system is increased during sleep.[12] The concentrations of various chemicals and hormones is quite different between day and night,[13] as is the activity of the liver.[14]

During wakefulness we are expending energy and breaking down body tissues, a process known as catabolism. Conversely, during sleep we are repairing our tissues, a process known as anabolism, hence the term anabolic steroids, which help to build up the durability of bones and the strength of muscles.

In all, more than a hundred biological functions have been shown to change in a manner dependant on whether it is day or night.[15]

It is clear, therefore, that sleep is not a period when we merely have our eyes closed and are oblivious to the outside world, but is instead a vastly different physiological state to wakefulness.

This unending rhythmicity of night and day, of sleep and wakefulness is known as the circadian or diurnal rhythm, and for practical purposes it is assumed to be a 24-hour cycle.

However, experiments were carried out in the 1930s in which subjects were placed in underground caves, in circumstances of near-perpetual darkness, and allowed to sleep or stay awake whenever they wished. Other experiments have been carried out exposing people to continuing light, such as that found within the Arctic circle during the summer months. In both cases all the subjects adjusted within time to a 25-hour clock! These experiments were subsequently refined in laboratory conditions and it was found that the natural inbuilt rhythmicity of the human clock is 24.8 hours.[16] How, therefore, do we keep to a 24-hour clock when our inbuilt clocks are attempting constantly to run on 24.8 hours?

The answer lies in a number of stimuli or cues that we receive from the outside world. These cues are known as *zeitgebers* (from the German for time-givers), of which the most important is light.

When light strikes the retina, in the back of each eye, signals are then carried through the brain to the occipital cortex at the back of the brain, thus allowing us to see what is going on around us.

However, some of these signals instead go to a different part of the brain, the supra chiasmatic nucleus (SCN), and thence to the pineal gland. This gland is about the size of a pea and is situated at the underside of the brain. When no signals are being brought to the pinéal gland from the retina it produces a hormone called melatonin. Conversely, when the retina is being stimulated by light and these signals are carried to the pineal gland it stops producing melatonin; i.e., the more darkness, the more melatonin; and vice versa.

There are other zeitgebers which are less important. For example, posture. Notice how easy it is to fall asleep when recumbent, even when reading an exciting book. By contrast, I have never known anyone to be able to stay asleep on their feet.

Noise too plays a part, it being easier to fall asleep when things are quiet, and increasingly difficult as the decibel level rises. Other possible zeitgebers include food, exercise, temperature, and level of general sensory input.

In conclusion, we each have an inbuilt clock which governs sleep and wakefulness, and which is set to run of its own accord at about 25 hours but is persuaded to stick to a 24-hour schedule by a number of outside stimuli called zeitgebers. And the hormone melatonin is the conductor that controls the orchestra of differences between what occurs in our bodies during sleep and during wakefulness.

All would therefore be well if, like our ancestors, we stayed put and slept and rose at approximately the same time each day.

2

The Flying Revolution

We live in a 24-hour world that does not sleep.

There was a time, perhaps as recently as the last century, when everybody slept by night and worked by day, but all that changed slowly but surely, decade by decade. We can perhaps blame Thomas Edison for this. Not only did he invent the electric light bulb but he himself despised sleep and regarded it largely as a waste of time and an indulgence of the lazy.[17] Doctors and nurses were required to be up at night, as disease and death are no respecters of time. Emergency services such as the fire brigade were required to be available on a 24-hour basis, as fires and other disasters could occur at any time. The police found it necessary to patrol by night in response to thieves who felt there were greater opportunities when workers from shops and factories were at home and in their beds.

Then two even bigger changes occurred which put an end to our previously more pastoral and tranquil way of life.

The first was the realization by factory owners that traditional work patterns left the valuable resource of their factories and foundries wasted for two thirds of the day, thus paving the way for the introduction of shift work.

The second big change was the coming of age of jet-powered air travel. In a global economy, for traders to trade they had to travel. In older days travel by ship or overland was sufficiently slow to allow one's inbuilt clock to adjust to new time zones as one went along. Modern jet travel using trans-polar routes allows one to be literally at the other end of the earth well within 24 hours, thus placing the inbuilt clock at complete loggerheads with its zeitgebers.

Nowadays very few people are unaffected by these changes. The highly successful chief executive of a successful multinational corporation is as likely to find his rhythms disturbed as the housewife who works shifts in a pea-processing factory.

Jetlag occurs whenever the normal circadian rhythm is disturbed. It tends to occur under two broad sets of circumstances.

The first occurs without our ever even leaving where we live, so the result is not strictly speaking jetlag, but we can still experience all the same symptoms. This situation arises with shift work, and particularly with a forward-rotating shift such as the following:

Day 1

> *Sleep:* midnight–0800 hrs
> *Work:* 0800–1600 hrs
> *Play:* 1600–2400 hrs

Day 2

> *Play:* midnight–0800 hrs
> *Sleep:* 0800–1600 hrs
> *Work:* 1600–2400 hrs

Day 3
   Work: midnight–0800 hrs
   Play: 0800–1600 hrs
   Sleep: 1600–2400 hrs

Day 4
   Sleep: midnight–0800 hrs
   Work: 0800–1600 hrs
   Play: 1600–2400 hrs . . .

Even the most stout-hearted of us will be a wreck within a week, and all because the day/night pattern will be completely out of phase with the inbuilt clock, and with no chance to catch up.

You don't have to be a factory shift worker to suffer these changes. The advent and exponential growth of information technology means that a trader in securities, commodities or currencies can now be in touch with what is going on all over the world at all times provided he or she is prepared to give up sleep altogether!

I have known patients prepared to set alarm clocks to let them tune in to closing prices in other markets at all hours of the night. The outcome has been inevitable. They may have had the edge when it came to trading but their health has suffered in the process.

The second (jetlag-proper) situation occurs when people are transported so rapidly across time zones that on arrival there has been no opportunity for their body clocks to catch up with the zeitgebers, or day/night cues, of their destinations. In the 19th century a journey from England to India would have taken many months to complete and there would have been ample time for the body clock to catch up and keep up as the journey progressed.

Nowadays such a distance could be covered in 8–9 hours, a blink of the eye by comparison.

This book is concerned with that second situation: true jetlag.

Imagine, for a moment, your own central-heating and hot-water control system at home. Typically it is timed to come on at 0700 hrs and go off at 0930, thus giving you heating, particularly in the winter, and hot water for your shower or bath. It stays off while you are out at work during the day and might come on again at 1800 hrs, giving you warmth for resting, cooking and washing, before it shuts off again at midnight, shortly after you have gone to bed.

Imagine now that you could suddenly transport your home to the other end of the world – a sort of 'Beam me up, Scottie' situation – and you did not adjust your controls to the new time zone. You would find no hot water in the morning when you got out of bed and the system would be on during the day, wasting energy. You might find no heating on arriving home in the evening, and it would come on while you were asleep, giving you a very restless night.

This is very similar to what happens to us when we travel through time zones.

3

Jetlag Vulnerability & Symptoms

What are the symptoms of jetlag and how do we know it is happening to us?

The best descriptions are vague and include a feeling of being 'not oneself' or 'out of sorts'. In normal good health one awakes in the morning feeling suitably refreshed and having a sense of energy and attack about the forthcoming day. We pause for some refreshment at lunchtime, which may make us feel like taking a short nap. There follows a second period of renewed energy, and as the day wears on we become contentedly fatigued. At 6–7 p.m. our capacity for creative work rapidly diminishes, but we are still receptive to passive activities such as watching T.V. A large meal is taken at between 7–10 p.m. and (unless we are 'owls') we feel pleasantly tired and ready for bed by 10–12 p.m.

Jetlag changes all of that, as follows:

The commonest symptom is inappropriate fatigue.[18] There is no sense of energy or enthusiasm on morning rising and one feels one is just 'going through the motions' of the day's activities. Some have described this to me as like trying to get through the day with a bad hangover. You feel tired, with an almost irresistible desire to sleep in the middle of the day. This is primarily due to sleep disturbance.[19] So common a problem is this that up to 80% of seasoned air crew report this type of disturbance during the first night after a long-haul flight. The figure is still up to 30% on the third night.[20] With these figures among the professionals, what hope has the relatively infrequent flier?

Worse still, the older you get, the more this becomes a problem.[21] Having got through the day you go to bed expecting a night's sleep – only to find sleep impossible or that, having got to sleep, you awake in the small hours completely unable to get back to sleep, but yet too tired to get up and do something productive.

And this fatigue is not merely mental. Accompanying it is physical fatigue. There is actually a decline in muscle strength and endurance after a long-haul flight.[22] The workout that is achieved effortlessly at home becomes so much more difficult in your host country's gym. Equally, the burst of energy that you get after a workout at home fails to materialize.

Accompanying this are disturbances in mood,[23] with irritability, disorientation, distortion of time and place and even confusion.[24] And these are not just subjective feelings. A whole host of psychological tests, carried out on volunteers undergoing intercontinental flight, have shown a large variety of mental impairments with jetlag.[25,26] You are not as alert, reaction time is increased and decision-making ability is reduced, to mention just a few. You may be irritated by your host colleagues' apparently poor performance, but in truth your own is probably much worse.

You can in fact test yourself on landing to see if jetlag has impaired your ability to perform. Kits for doing this are available from the Jetlag Clinic. (See page 119 for contact details.) It might be wise, if such testing reveals significant impairment, to delegate to a colleague or postpone a meeting until you can demonstrate that you have picked up.

Driving should also be avoided whilst you are mentally impaired by jetlag.

The gastrointestinal system becomes particularly upset. A common complaint is of hunger at odd times of the day and night.[27] Another is that sitting down to lunch or dinner is not accompanied by expected appetite. The bowels become irregular, and those fortunate enough not to catch gastroenteritis due to eating or drinking infected food or water usually become constipated. In addition, heartburn, nausea and abdominal discomfort are all more common after flying long-haul.[28]

Women flying across time zones are prone to problems with periods. When flying on a regular basis, for example as cabin attendants, they are more likely to suffer from irregular cycles[29] and more painful periods.[30]

Aches and pains arising from muscles and joints become more frequent and severe.[31]

The manner in which the kidneys cope with waste products and eliminate them from the body in the urine becomes disordered.[32] Toxic waste products can build up in the body as a result. A whole host of metabolic processes that normally occur in a rhythmic manner become seriously upset.[33] The cumulative effect of all these changes is to increase the amount of stress we are exposed to[34] – as if we were not already exposed to enough in our daily working lives.

If all these symptoms, and the terrible things that happen to you when you experience jetlag, are beginning to sound like some dread disease – good! It is about time that people – especially the people who are sending you around the world in the first place – woke up to the fact that jetlag is not to be taken lightly.

Who suffers and how badly?

Not surprisingly, as with everything else in life, there is a wide variation in how badly people suffer. As an approximation, roughly 25% of people have little or no difficulty adapting, 25% have severe problems with jetlag and the remaining 50% are somewhere in between.[35]

Are there factors which can help you guess beforehand whether you are likely to suffer badly from jetlag?

There certainly are. Let's look at some of the individual traits that determine this likelihood.

Take *rhythm stability* first. The more rigid your 24-hour rhythm, the more likely you are to suffer from jetlag.[36] The stability of your rhythm can be worked out by taking your temperature (accurately with a mercury thermometer!) several times throughout the day, and if possible with the assistance of a partner once or twice during the night. The graph showing your body temperature should look something like this:

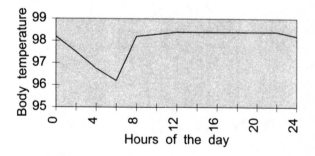

So if you find that the highs and lows of your temperature occur at exactly the same time, day after day, and your chart repeats itself exactly, time after time, you have a very rigid cycle. If on the other hand the time when your temperature is at its highest or lowest is variable, then you have a more labile or fluid cycle and are therefore less likely to suffer from jetlag.

Next is the so-called *amplitude* of your rhythm. This is the measure of the difference between your highest and lowest temperatures. You simply subtract your lowest temperature from your highest and this gives you the amplitude. The graphs below show two individuals. One with a high amplitude; high = 98.4, low = 96.2, so amplitude = 2.2. Like this:

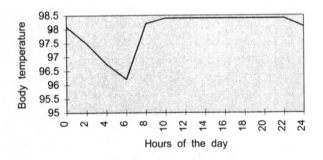

And the second with a low amplitude; high = 98.3, low = 96.6, so amplitude = 1.7. Like this:

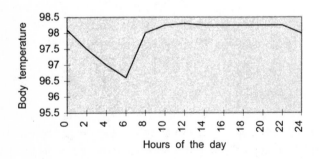

The higher your amplitude, the less likely you are to suffer from jetlag.[37]

Age is also important.

The ability to withstand changes to the body clock declines as we get older and it takes us longer to adapt.[38]

The more rigid our *sleep patterns* are, the more likely we are to suffer. If you are someone who simply *has* to be in bed by 11 p.m. and *has* to get up at 7 a.m., and who feels shattered the following day if your pattern is disturbed, you will fare less well.[39]

So-called owls tend to be less affected than larks.[40]

Personality type also matters.

The more extroverted you are, the more rapidly you adapt.[41] (Kits to determine how susceptible you are to jetlag are available from the Jetlag Clinic. See page 119.)

If you are reading this book and wondering what all the fuss is all about, relax! You are in the top 25%. Equally well, if you are a major sufferer, take heart: you are not alone.

How dangerous is jetlag?

Some believe not at all and point to the fact that by 1984 three women and over 150 men had spent periods of up to 185 consecutive days in space without apparent ill effect.[42] However, others point to the more insidious effects of long-term exposure to jetlag. There is certainly an increased incidence of heart disease amongst shift workers, compared with their peers who work only by day.[43] Overall mortality figures are also higher amongst shift workers.[44]

And yet if we consider the health of those exposed most to jetlag, i.e. the airline pilots, they do not seem to do too badly. Pilots who spend a great deal of their lives in a jetlag fug are far less likely to die from most causes of death – except air crashes – at any particular age than the rest of us.[45] Interestingly, however, one noticeable cause of natural death that pilots are more likely to die from is brain tumours, which raises the question whether frequent fliers of all professions may be exposed to greater risk for this condition. No doubt this possibility will be explored by researchers in due course.

4

Some Statistics

How common is the problem?

Well, let's look at some statistics. The International Air Transport Association publishes statistics on an annual basis. Let's look at some of these for 1996 (the latest figures available at time of going to press).[46]

The world's busiest airports are O'Hare at Chicago, Hartsfield in Atlanta, and Fort Worth in Dallas. But the greater majority of the passengers using these airports are domestic, commuting between various U.S. cities and not therefore generally subject to jetlag.

The fourth busiest airport in the world is London Heathrow. In 1996 it reported throughput in excess of 54 million passengers travelling through it, of whom over 46 million were international passengers: more than two thirds of the entire U.K. population.

A staggering 371 million passengers were carried internationally in this year, but of course not all of these flights would have involved travel that could inflict *serious* jetlag. So let's now focus on some of the flights that would have had a greater propensity to induce jetlag.

Over 28 million passengers travelled from North America to Europe or back. Just over 2 million passengers travelled between Heathrow and JFK New York alone in this year.[47] There were over 14.5 million passengers travelling from North America to Asia or back. In addition, over 15 million passengers travelled from Europe to Asia or back, together with 2 million people going from Europe to Southwest Pacific or back. Thus, at a very minimum in 1996, we had 60 million journeys likely to cause jetlag. And these figures are set to rise.

For example, in April 1996 the British Airports Authority reported that in the previous month the number of people travelling through its airports had risen to 7.7 million, up 11% on March 1995.[48]

Many readers of this book will recall some business mistakes they have made. Big business is understandably reluctant to publish or indeed discuss such cases. However, some figures are available from studies done. One survey has shown that on arriving at their destination 50% of businessmen were required to conduct business meetings *before* they had the benefit of a night's sleep. Less than 20% of the total felt that they were fit to hold their meetings at the appointed time.[49] We can also find examples of jetlag resulting in serious consequences for figures famous enough to make the world's headlines.

Even presidents of the USA are not exempt. President George Bush took sleeping pills to help him cope with jetlag. People do not normally experience problems with their speech patterns due to sleeping pills. But the combination of jetlag and pills was too much for someone even with the stamina of an ex boss of the CIA. Bush's job as President would obviously not allow him to give up the travelling, so the pills had to go.[50]

And Boris Yeltsin! A man well able to handle his drink at home, in the fine Russian tradition, he found that when alcohol combined with jetlag his speech became slurred,[51] and on landing in Ireland it all caught up with him to the extent that he was unable to get off his plane to meet the host president.

In the 1950s the then U.S. Secretary of State, John Foster Dulles, flew to Egypt to negotiate the Aswan Dam treaty. He arrived fatigued and irritable from jetlag. The result? A botched diplomatic job, and the project going to the Soviets.[52]

During 1982 another U.S. Secretary of State, Alexander M. Haig, was attempting to mediate between Britain and Argentina to avoid war in the Falkland Islands. In one two-week period he flew 30,000 miles. In one eight-day period he would have had to change his watch 22 times to a different time zone.[53] And what happened?

The Falklands War was not avoided.

When such mishaps, failure and embarrassment befall some of the world's toughest and most capable men and women, due to jetlag, who else is likely to survive it without help?

5

Adverse Effects of Flying

In addition to the problems of jetlag itself, there are other factors which lead to a decline in human performance. The only way to travel fast enough to get jetlag is by the modern jet aircraft and travelling in these produces its own unique set of problems which make jetlag worse.

The opulence of the first- and business-class cabins belies the fact that at cruising altitudes, say 35,000 ft, the atmosphere outside is so inhospitable that it cannot support any form of life. Indeed, without the oxygen which is supplied from overhead masks in the case of sudden decompression – if, say, the aircraft were to develop a leak – exposure to the high-altitude environment would produce unconsciousness in a matter of seconds and death within minutes.

In an ideal world the oxygen in the cabin would be continuously of the same concentration as that at sea level. Yet if one were to achieve that by travelling just a few hundred feet above ground, in the manner say of a helicopter, the resistance produced by the air to forward movement would be so great that speed would be greatly reduced. Worse, the fuel tanks would soon be empty, and you would have to keep putting down every few hundred miles to refuel, thus defeating the whole purpose of air travel and making trans-Atlantic flight impossible.

And, as we have seen, to fly at 35,000 ft without supplemental oxygen, our planes could carry only cargo and would have to be flown by robots, since human life could not survive.

We operate therefore by compromise: the cabin is partially pressurized. Typically this pressurization is to the equivalent of an altitude of 8000 ft. – i.e., when actually cruising at 35–40,000 ft we are exposed to the same air pressure as if we were standing on top of a mountain 8000 ft high. The exact figures vary from aircraft to aircraft. For example, whereas the McDonnell Douglas DC-9 simulates an altitude of 8000 ft,[54] the Boeing 747 simulates a considerably lower altitude of about 4700 ft. The timetables of most airlines specify which aircraft are flown on each flight, so you can deliberately and in advance book flights on aircraft which simulate lower altitudes, this being preferable where possible.

Travelling ·under these simulated circumstances, no matter what the altitude equivalent, produces a number of specific problems for all jet-flight travellers.

Oxygen shortage

As there is a decrease in the amount of oxygen available in the air, there is a decline in the amount of oxygen circulating in the blood. This in turn leads to less oxygen reaching the tissues of the body and in particular the brain, which is particularly sensitive to decreases in available oxygen. This decrease in available oxygen is called hypoxia.

Hypoxia becomes a problem for some people at about 5000 ft but affects most people at 8000 ft.[55] And this is exactly the effective operating range of altitude of most jets. The changes that occur due to hypoxia are slow and subtle and unless you are aware of these possible changes in your functioning you will have no insight into what is happening or else you may incorrectly attribute these changes to other causes.

First comes a mild euphoria, a feeling of release, of a weight being lifted from you – especially if the plane has to fly through cloud before emerging to a bright blue sky filled with sunlight.

This is followed by behavioural changes. We have all seen passengers who on boarding seem pleasant and mild-mannered, but a few hours into the flight can get picky and irritable. Others become disinhibited, especially if assisted by alcohol, and do things they would never do on terra firma, such as flirting outrageously with air hostesses.

Next comes memory impairment and loss of judgement.

Finally come mental and muscular inco-ordination.

There are other, further effects of hypoxia but unless you have a very bad pair of lungs you are unlikely to encounter these at the equivalent of 8000 ft.

The euphoria is generally harmless and the dangers of disinhibition are self-evident. Resist the temptation to open up and tell your boss what's wrong with the way he is running the business!

The memory loss and decline in judgement are more serious matters. Many business travellers, especially those armed with laptop computers, regard their aircraft seat as an office away from the office. This is fine so long as you realize the mental constraints.

The problem lies not so much in doing things that are familiar, but in coping with new situations.[56]

This is why pilots spend so much of their training time working in simulators and thereafter, throughout their careers, regularly updating themselves in them. This way they learn how to deal with all possible situations as if they were routine. And so, when they encounter a genuine emergency situation in the air, hypoxia will not effect their decision-making processes as they are not dealing with a 'new' situation. For them it is routine.

For you, however, as passenger, and particularly if you are flying on business, there are important practical implications.

It is perfectly all right, for example, to rehearse an already-laid-out presentation, but you would be ill-advised to plan one from scratch. Okay, say, to go through your expense receipts, but not to plan the operating strategy for your department for the next twelve months.

It is all right to read new material but you will notice that it can take longer to absorb. It's also a bit more difficult to recall it later. The message is clear: stick to the familiar, to the already planned out. Do not use a jet flight to plan new projects.[57] Remember that this effect of hypoxia on thinking processes is made considerably worse by jetlag, so that what you might just manage going London-to-J'burg you will not get away with on a Berlin-to-Singapore flight.

Hyperventilation

This literally means overbreathing. Many people when they breathe air which is thin and dry, particularly if they are of an anxious disposition, get a vague feeling of suffocation, a feeling that they are not getting enough air in, and so they start to overbreathe. As they do so, they get more oxygen in but they also get rid of more carbon dioxide, the waste product we dump while breathing.

Carbon dioxide determines the acidity in our bodies and, for complex physiological reasons, when we dump more than we should we lose acidity. This produces a feeling of lightheadedness and unreality. If you continue overbreathing you then get pins and needles in your fingers followed by muscular spasms and twitches. Eventually panic supervenes, followed by loss of consciousness. This, surprisingly, is not as dangerous as it sounds. Having lost consciousness, you simply revert to breathing normally, and before long you wake up. You can get a feeling of what hyperventilation is like by deliberately taking half a dozen deep breaths. This is far short of what is required to make you pass out.

The traditional treatment for hyperventilation is to rebreathe your own air via a brown paper bag. This, however, has the disadvantage of looking rather ridiculous. Breathing exercises are more effective and are not likely to be noticed by your fellow passengers. You take a deep breath in over a slow count to four. Continuing the count, hold the breath in until you get to twelve, then let it out over thirteen to sixteen. Stop and wait till you feel you want to take another breath, then repeat the exercise. This will give you control over your breathing without upsetting your acidity.

Dehydration and effects of recycled air

The air that you breathe in an aircraft is brought in from the outside atmosphere by the aircraft's engines. As it comes in it is cooled, and, unfortunately, whatever little water vapour there is at cruising altitude is removed in the process. As a result, the cabin air is drier than any of the world's deserts. Relative humidity (the amount of moisture in the air) is typically 20% in the Sahara desert. Optimum comfort is obtained at about 50%. But in a jet, as the flight progresses the humidity gradually falls until, by the end of a long-haul flight, it can be as low as 1%.[58]

Why, you ask, don't airlines humidify the air and give us all an easier time. The answer is cost. Air can be humidified only by water. Apart from the cost of necessary hardware, an average Boeing 747 would need 2200 lbs of water for a typical flight. This equates to about 15 passengers who could not be carried.[59]

Many of the older planes, built before 1985, provided 100% fresh air which was completely changed every three minutes. In order to reduce fuel costs involved in the process of cooling the air delivered to the ventilation systems, from the engines, more recent aircraft produce an equal measure of fresh and recirculated air, which is changed every 6–7 minutes. Moreover, ventilation rates differ depending which part of the aircraft you are in. The cockpit, where the pilots are, may well receive 100% fresh air, the reason being that eyesight, particularly at night, is very sensitive to a fall in oxygen.[60] It wouldn't do for them not to be able to read their instruments! The ventilation in the first-class cabin is typically three times better than that in the economy section. On an average flight, ventilation rate for your pilot is typically ten times higher than that for the economy passenger.[61]

The practical consequences of this situation are two-fold. First, in re-breathing other people's air you are also inhaling their germs, making you much more susceptible to developing infections, particularly infections of the respiratory tract.[62] Unfortunately, the wearing of masks, goggles, etc, does nothing to alleviate the effects of recycled air.

There is not much you can do during a flight to alleviate this problem. However, where practicable you should avoid flying when tired, run down or overworked, since your immune system is then at its lowest ebb. (Show this paragraph to your boss!) Likewise, avoid flying immediately following a bereavement, a divorce, or even uprooting and moving home, as all of these can have a depressant effect on the immune system.

Secondly, inhaling so much extremely dry air has a damaging effect on the eyes and respiratory passages. Have you noticed how pink or even red the whites of your eyes look immediately on alighting from an aircraft – even if you haven't been drinking. Susceptible people complain of dry, itchy eyes. This can be overcome by using artificial tears such as Hypromellose eye drops, which can normally be bought from a chemist without prescription.

More severe cases may need combination drops containing steroids and antibiotics (e.g., Betamethazone / Neomycin; prescription needed) before embarking on a particularly long flight.

The dry air often causes crusting and discomfort in the nose. Again, this is overcome by using specialized nasal drops. Brand-name drops, such as Ocean, Ayr or Nasal, can be purchased as above, without prescription.

The inner airways from the throat down to the lungs need to be kept adequately hydrated during long flights. This can be achieved by keeping a glass or cup of liquid on your table. The surrounding air is so dry that this liquid evaporates rapidly and moistens the air in much the same way that some people keep a saucer of water near their central heating radiator to prevent the air getting too dry at home.

Another option is to hold on to the hot towel you are given after your meal. While this is still wet and warm, tip your head back and place the towel over your face. Breathe normally. When it dries out, replenish from time to time with hot water provided by the cabin crew, using the same source used to make tea and coffee. The hot water in the toilets, though clean enough for washing your hands, is not sterile enough to inhale.

It is also vital to protect all the other tissues of your body from dehydration on long flights by ensuring an adequate intake of fluids, but be aware of the effects of alcohol and fizzy drinks, as discussed below.

Despite the annoyance and inconvenience of such flight effects on your respiratory passages, it is cheering to know that you are unlikely to suffer serious harm. Airline pilots, the people who have to endure this all the time, are actually less likely to die from respiratory diseases than us normal mortals![63]

Gas expansion

As the pressure outside your body decreases with ascent, gas inside your body expands. There is a considerable amount of gas inside the intestines. Expansion of this gas will produce a sensation of bloating and distension and in severe cases will produce abdominal discomfort or even pain. Anyone who easily suffers from this problem, and it does vary from person to person, should avoid drinking fizzy drinks for 24 hours before and also during a flight (enough time to let the gas work its way through) and avoid certain foods which are known to produce extra gas in the intestines, e.g., beans, cabbage, Brussels sprouts and turnips.

Ascent and descent also produce changes in the volume and pressure of gases contained in the sinuses and ears, with important practical consequences. During ascent the air contained in the middle-ear cavity and the sinuses will expand, pushing outward and causing a painful rise in pressure – unless it can be equalized with the pressure of the air outside the head. This is easily accomplished by swallowing or yawning. Small babies don't realize this and hence their crying during ascent and descent which 'mysteriously' disappears once the plane has levelled out.

Be warned that if you fly with a heavy head cold, then yawning, swallowing, blowing with a pinched nose, and so on, will be unable to equalize these gas pressures and the result will be very painful. You can even suffer ruptured ear drums if ascent or descent is too rapid. This painful damage to the ear drums is known as barotrauma. If the boss insists on your flying with such a head cold (despite having been shown this book!) it is very important to prepare yourself with adequate doses of decongestants, antihistamines, nasal drops, etc.

Mobility

You are pretty well stuck in your seat for the duration of the flight – unless you do something about it. Even though the immobility suffered in first class is a great deal more comfortable than that endured in economy, the basic problems remain the same.

Joints that are not regularly put through their full range of movement become stiff and painful. Piles (haemorrhoids, or 'judge's bum') become worse and there is a danger that the blood in the lower legs will clot and produce a thrombosis.[64] The solution is obvious. You either make use of the long aisle space and walk up and down from time to time (that's why an aisle seat is often the best one to book) or use inflight exercises without leaving your seat. Instructions for these exercises are often found at the back of the in-flight magazine.

Cancer

Fly for long enough, as the airline pilots themselves do, and your chances of getting cancer of the prostate, brain cancer, malignant melanoma (a skin cancer) or leukaemia are all greatly increased. The better news, strangely, is that the risk of getting cancer overall is significantly reduced by spending long hours in the sky.[65]

In summary, there are a number of irritating, uncomfortable and even potentially serious hazards awaiting the long-distance traveller *before* he or she has to tackle the problems of jetlag. No one regime works for everybody, and most travellers find their own personally tailored solutions through trial and error. Observe the guidelines in this chapter, and your learning curve should be smoother.

6

The Strategies

So we now understand that jetlag is a highly unpleasant condition that arises when our inbuilt 24-hour body clock is sending us one set of signals which contradicts the signals that we are getting from the outside world.

The fundamental strategy for avoiding jetlag can be summarized as follows:

- *If possible, avoid having to adjust your body clock at all.*

- *Any unavoidable adjustment should be accomplished as rapidly and decisively as possible.*

1. SHORT JOURNEYS

The average person experiences few or no symptoms of jetlag if asked to make an adjustment of up to two hours time-zone difference on either side. This means that, for example, someone normally resident in Cairo can fly east to Karachi or west to Madrid without experiencing any symptoms.

However, as explained in Chapter 1, the inbuilt clock is always trying to assert a 25-hour rhythm (the 24-hour cycle being imposed by virtue of a 24-hour day/night pattern). When you fly east you 'lose' time and your day becomes shorter. By flying west you 'gain' time and your day becomes longer. As your own clock is already trying to lengthen your day, you are working with your body. This explains why everybody suffers much more when flying east.[66]

You therefore have a little more leeway when flying west, so that the 'safe zone' within which you can reliably expect no problems is two time zones eastward and up to three time zones westward. The less rigid your inbuilt clock, the more latitude you will have with this.

Thus the traveller heading east from London should have no problems flying to Berlin or Moscow, but might expect problems going further – to Muscat, say, or beyond.

West from London (beyond England) there are no significant land masses within three time zones, other than parts of Brazil. Flying to New York involves five time zones, and this, as we all know, produces problems.

When making such journeys, *do nothing to your clock!* On departure, just set your watch (preferably your second watch – see below) to destination time, and otherwise carry on as usual.

2. 'IN&OUT TRIPS'

Because it takes several days normally to adjust to a new time zone, it is practical and indeed desirable, in a number of circumstances, to leave your body clock set to home time.

This happens most commonly when a businessman is required to make one trip for a meeting lasting perhaps one to two hours but where the flight is more than two zones eastward or three zones westward. Common examples include the New York/London run, Paris/Bombay or Tokyo/Los Angeles.

But what happens in practice?

Typically, your secretary or travel agency will make

arrangements to fly you out to arrive 12–18 hours before your meeting, so you can 'settle in' first. They may then allow another 12–18 hours after the meeting for you to wind down before flying back.

Nothing could be worse!

Seriously, nothing flies more in the face of what we know about circadian physiology than that approach. You will have started to adjust to the new time zone during those first 12–18 hours. Then you are abruptly dropped back to where you were to begin with – a sort of double jetlag!

Far better to adopt what I call the In&Out tactic, which works as follows: you get straight in and have your meeting, then you get straight out again, all the time keeping your body clock on home time. Let's look at some examples.

You are an investment banker based in New York, and you are required to fly to London for a four-hour meeting. You catch the BA116 flight from JFK at 2220 hrs. You eat dinner at home or at the airport before departure and immediately on boarding the plane you indicate to the cabin crew that you wish to sleep right through. You get off to sleep as fast as you can. Alcohol and sleeping pills should be avoided due to the short flying time and early start the following day.

You arrive the following morning at 1005 hrs, London time. This is equivalent to 0505 your time, so you are having an early start but nothing you cannot handle. You have scheduled your meeting for, say, 1300 hrs London time. This is 0800 for you, so you will have occupied yourself by having your usual breakfast between landing and the meeting. You will have politely declined lunch and especially alcohol before this meeting. You head straight for the airport following the meeting to catch

BA179, departing at 1830 hrs. As this is 1330 by your body clock you can enjoy a leisurely lunch on board, and perhaps even a congratulatory drink, as you will be arriving in JFK at 2135 hrs and home in time for dinner. Thereafter you should have no difficulty sleeping through the night. This is because you have not shifted your clock.

Now imagine you are an advertising executive living in London and have to fly to Abu Dhabi to give a three-hour presentation. You catch the Gulf Airways flight GF008, departing from Heathrow at 2215 hrs and arriving in Abu Dhabi at 0910 local time the following morning. Businesses have already opened for the day in this part of the world. You go directly to your meeting, make your presentation and arrive back at Abu Dhabi airport in plenty of time to catch the Emirates flight EK005 at 1420 hrs, arriving back in London at 1830 – there being no suitable Gulf Air or British Airways flight to accomplish this return journey. It is worth noting too that Emirates do not have a suitable outbound flight, their nearest being EK006, which departs LHR at 2000 hrs on Wednesdays only. This illustrates the principle that to successfully overcome jetlag you must be prepared to split airlines occasionally.

Because London is four hours behind Abu Dhabi it will be 1820, London time, when you board the return flight. You can therefore celebrate the brilliance of your presentation with a drink, arrive back in time to take in a movie or a show, have dinner and be home in bed at your usual time. All the time you keep your watch on London time and eat your meals when you normally would.

Next consider the Hong Kong businessman who needs to fly to Auckland in New Zealand to meet with potential new partners and to sign a deal. Auckland is four hours

ahead. He takes the Cathay Pacific CX107, departing
at 2110 hrs Hong Kong time, arriving at 1240 local
time in Auckland the following day. This will be 0730
by his body clock, so time to get up anyway, having enjoyed a good meal and a decent seven hours
sleep on board. He has an hour or so to meet these
people at the airport, sign the papers and catch the
Cathay Pacific CX108 non-stop flight departing from
Auckland at 1410 hrs local time and arriving at 2010,
local time in Hong Kong. If the meeting runs over-
time – and if it's a Thursday! – he can always catch
the Air New Zealand flight NZ79, departing Auckland
at 1455 hrs and getting him home by 2055 hrs, Hong
Kong time.

Those are just a few of many possible examples. The
important thing to remember is that this sort of flight
planning is much better for you as you have to make
no adaptation to time zones. If you are self-employed
you can make your own arrangements to take this advice
into account. If on the other you work for a merchant
bank, advertising agency or management consultancy,
you should insist that the travel department in your
company makes the arrangements to suit you. Apart
from the advantages of less jetlag, and therefore a more
successful business trip, the time you would have spent
'settling in' and 'winding down' can now be spent either
in the office getting some real work done or else relaxing
with your family.

3. 'I'M STILL AT HOME' FLIGHTS

A further type of In&Out situation arises when you are
forced to stay in your destination for 2–3 days, but where
it is still possible to stay on home time. I call these the
'I'm-still-at-home' flights.

The classic example is the Londoner going to New York for the weekend, or vice versa.

Timing of flights here is less critical as you are going to be there for 2–3 days in any case. Do, however, remember to time the outbound flight so as not to interfere with your night's sleep the night before departure. So, for example, do not depart from Heathrow at 0600 hrs when taking a weekend trip to New York. If you are heading off on a Friday you will have ruined Thursday night's sleep and begun to shift your body clock into a different and contrary time zone. (If you are used to getting out of bed at say 0730 hrs each morning and you then have to rise at 0330 for this 0600 flight you will, by getting up four hours earlier, be shifting your clock forward – i.e., eastward, on a morning when you are flying westward!)

If anything, you want to take a late-morning flight to edge your clock just a little bit westward by staying asleep a little longer.

The choice is wide. You can take the United Airlines flight UA907, departing from LHR at 1335 hrs and arriving at Newark at 1630. If you prefer Gatwick for your departure, there is Continental Airlines flight CO25, departing at 1100 hrs and arriving at Newark at 1400.

Ideally, you take two watches with you, and on arrival at New York you do two things:

First, adjust one watch to New York time. This is to ensure that you are not late for appointments. Your second watch you keep on London time.

You then go about your day (and night) according to London time. Accordingly, you go to bed at about 1900 hrs, NY time, and rise at 0300. This is eminently possible in the 'city that doesn't sleep', to quote Frank Sinatra. It may be somewhat more difficult to do this in the dead of winter, when it is dark on rising, but it should be a lot easier in summer.

Business meetings should be held at 7 a.m., New York time, which is equivalent to 12 midday London time: when you are at the peak of your mental fitness. Fortunately, such breakfast meetings are very popular in the U.S. You should avoid negotiating from approximately 0830–1000, NY time, as you will (or should) then be having your lunch and this will produce a slight rise in melatonin levels and a consequent drowsiness, with decreased vigilance and concentration (unless you are an avid owl). Lunch should be followed by a brisk walk, there being daylight at this time even in winter. You can rejoin the fray at 1000 hrs, NY time, and you will be good for another 4–5 hours minimum. Do not allow talks to spill over beyond 1700 hrs local time as your body clock will now be on 2200 hrs (London time) and you will be getting tired and less sharp in your concentration.

Breakfast, lunch and dinner should be eaten at the time you would normally eat them in London. New York is a 24-hour city and there is no difficulty obtaining dinner there at 1600 hrs, local time, or breakfast at 0300.

Your body clock will try to adjust to the time cues that it is given in terms of getting out of and going back to bed, darkness and light, timing of meals, etc. It is therefore vital to keep as many of these cues as possible on your London time. Ideally, all of them. So, for example, you should ensure that from 1700 hrs NY time you avoid blazing sunshine. Wear sunglasses when outside – many people do so in NY anyway. When indoors sit in dim surroundings and when going to bed at 1900 hrs, local time, ensure that your room is totally dark. You should have no difficulty going off to sleep as it is now midnight in London. Conversely, when your alarm clock wakes you at 0300 hrs, local time, you should flood your room with as much bright light as possible and go out to eat breakfast in the loudest most garish restaurant you can find. In this situation you will find the light mask or the 1000 watt lamp very helpful.

Similar trips include Rio/LA, Bahrain/Bangkok and Delhi/Tokyo. Exactly the same principles apply to a 2–3 day stopover in any other city. Take two watches and stick to your home time. Note, however, that this strategy becomes progressively more difficult to put into operation the less cosmopolitan your destination. Try getting breakfast at four o'clock in the morning in Nairobi or Reykjavik, and you may be in for a disappointment.

One of the pioneers of the I'm-still-at-home approach was President Lyndon Johnson. When travelling long distance he would keep his watch on Washington Time, eating and sleeping accordingly. His reason? 'Jetlag gives me indigestion and I won't put up with it!' He was equally dismissive of any objections to his approach. 'They can go to bed a few hours later if they want to talk to the President of the United States.'

4. FLYING WEST IS BEST

Because the 24-hour cycle is constantly trying to stretch to 25 when left to its own devices, scientists have been looking at the practical consequences of this. They have taken groups of healthy volunteers and brought them halfway round the world, some in an easterly direction and others west. The volunteers were then asked to rate their jetlag symptoms on a daily basis. In all cases the suffering was far worse when travelling east.

In addition it took longer to recover after flying east-ward – on average 8-9 days, as opposed to 4–5 days recovery time after flying west.[67]

Therefore, when taking a business trip that involves a number of destinations around the world before returning to your home base, always travel westward for the meetings and eastward coming home. You will be in better shape for the meetings and you can then recover at home when the pressure is off. If your trip involves half or more of the circumference of the earth – i.e., 12 or more time zones, carry on flying the way you are so as to arrive back home from the east. The New York businessman conducting meetings in Los Angeles, Hong Kong and Bombay, with a last one in Berlin, should go home travelling west from to Berlin to New York. Passengers undertaking round-the-world holidays, or who have a series of meetings in different destinations around the world, ending up at their original point of departure, should insist on flying westward. This applies particularly to politicians engaged in 'shuttle diplomacy'. Schedule your meetings in the order of (e.g.) London, Washington, Tokyo, Delhi, Cairo, Paris, London.

Avoid (e.g.) London, Madrid, Moscow, Karachi, Peking, Bogota, London.

5. 'VERTICAL FLIGHTS'

Finally we come to the special case of so-called vertical flights. These are long-haul north/south or south/north flights. How, you may ask, could they possibly cause jetlag when we aren't even changing time zones?

The answer lies back in Chapter 2, where I explained that it was possible to suffer the equivalent of jetlag without ever leaving home: by adversely affecting one's sleep schedule.

Examples would include Toronto/Montevideo, London/Johannesburg, and Tokyo/Sydney. The traveller undertaking such 'vertical' flights is at risk of developing a jetlag-like syndrome unless caution is exercised as follows:

Let us say you are flying London to Johannesburg, or New York to Buenos Aires. Each of these flights takes approximately 12 hours and both involve virtually no change of time zone. Imagine that each flight departs at 0800 hrs local time and arrives therefore at about 2000 hrs (being in the same time zone, no clock change is necessary). By departing at 0800 hrs you probably have to get out of bed at about 0500 hrs, so that's one night's sleep down the drain for a start. By the time you clear Customs, find your way to your hotel, check in, and have something to eat and drink, it may well be after midnight. So if you have an early start in the morning you have another night's sleep cut short. The alternative is to sleep in, but by doing this you are shifting your time clock backwards in a westerly direction.

Similarly, if you caught a flight that left at 1800 hrs you would not lose sleep the night before the flight, but by arriving at 0600 hrs you would interrupt your sleep for *that* night, as you would be getting up earlier than normal and therefore shifting your clock forward in an easterly direction.

It's best to plan these 'vertical' flights so as to avoid changing the time that you would normally rise and go to bed. I would therefore take flight BA55, departing Heathrow at 2145 hrs and arriving in Johannesburg at 1040 hrs – in preference to BA61 (which arrives at 0550 hrs) or South African Airways flight SA235 (arriving at 0720).

7

Switching the Clock

We now come to a discussion of those flights which involve a shift of time zone of more than 6–7 hours and/or where you are required to stop over for more than 2–3 days.

With these flights a different strategy has to be employed. This is because:

1 The pressure on your clock to change becomes much stronger after six time zones.

2 The amount of mutually suitable time for meeting becomes substantially less. Thus, In&Out meetings become less feasible.

Accordingly, in this situation, *you have to adapt your body clock to that of your destination*. And you should make the change to the new time zone as EARLY as possible and as RAPIDLY as possible. These are two entirely different requirements and both must be put into effect.

The early changes

Don't wait until you have arrived at your destination to switch either your watch or your body clock to the local time. Make the change before you board the plane and even as early as the night before. You should therefore

avoid flights which depart at a time that corresponds
to the middle of the night in terms of the destination
time zone. This is most easily explained by an example.
Suppose you are flying from London to Singapore at a
time of year when Singapore is eight hours ahead of
London. If you get on a plane at Heathrow at 1900 hrs,
you will of necessity be awake! Meanwhile it is 0300 hrs
in Singapore, and sensible people will be in their beds. If
you are attempting an early adaptation to Singapore time
you too should be asleep. As explained in Chapter 6,
adaptation will take a certain length of time. So the
sooner you start to change, the sooner the adaptation
occurs. You should therefore endeavour to take a flight
that departs London between 2400 and 1600 hrs London
time (= 0800–2400 hrs Singapore time), so that you are
awake when everyone in Singapore is awake.

The rapid changes

As explained in Chapter 1, the body clock is con-
strained, programmed by a number of stimuli called
zeitgebers. Working from the strongest to the weakest,
they include: light and darkness (with its consequent
Melatonin secretion), sleep and wakefulness, timing of
food and meals, sociability, posture, exercise, excitement
and tranquillity.

The more of these factors that are brought into play
before you depart the better. So start thinking and acting
according to destination time before you actually leave.
This will get the ball rolling so that the time taken to fully
adapt on arrival is reduced.

Chapter 14, 'Practical Flight Management', shows in
some detail how our general strategy can be effectively
implemented for three of the most commonly undertaken
long-distance flights; two east and one west. The actual

flights shown (subject to timetable changes) are amongst the best to take in terms of training your clock as you go. Very often there are similar flights with other airlines which will be just as good.

Not uncommonly, though, there is no ideally suitable flight from a jetlag-avoidance point of view. It is unfortunate that many airlines and the regulators have not woken up to the fact that it is in no-one's interest to be getting on a plane at half past four in the morning, destination time. However, even where none of the available flights is ideal, or if your own schedule will not allow you to book the best flight available for the trip, it is still possible to prepare and programme yourself to make the most of the situation: all with a view to minimizing any jetlag effects you might suffer.

Some flights on some routes will involve you in getting on a plane in the early morning, destination time, and sleeping for a variable period. E.g., Frankfurt/Toronto or Seoul/Amsterdam. When you get out of bed on the morning of such a flight you should do so as quietly as possible and keep yourself on night mode – dim lights, postponing breakfast, etc – until it is time to wake up on such a flight. Always bear in mind that it is the local time at destination which you are trying to shift to. Our assumption for the statistically average passenger is that he or she will normally sleep eight hours per night and do so between midnight and 8 a.m. If you are a lark, you should bring these times back, to compensate, and if you are an owl you should advance them correspondingly.

And so on.

An exhaustive list of the best flights to take, from the point of view of beating jetlag, would be too long to include in this book. Specific help, and personalized flight programmes in accordance with the author's advice, can be obtained from the Jetlag Clinic. Please refer to the final page of this book for contact details.

8

To Sleep, To Wake

In Chapter 7 we saw how to plan picking the right flights and staying awake or sleeping in order to accelerate the change in your body clock to that of your destination.

Having arrived at your destination, you must continue the process of changing your body clock to local time as quickly and determinedly as possible. This may well involve staying awake when you really want to sleep, or sleeping when your clock is telling you to stay awake. Special tactics have to be employed, therefore, to achieve your objective.

It helps at this stage to decide whether you are the sort of person who can sleep easily on command or whether you find that you can stay awake without too much difficulty for long periods without seemingly adversely affecting your alertness and mental capabilities. This is an entirely different concept from Larks v. Owls as discussed earlier. One owl can' easily have a nap after lunch; another cannot sleep at all during the day. Some professions seem to train you for one or the other. Hospital doctors, such as surgeons in training, learn to stay awake for very long hours without a break, whereas in the armed forces you learn to grab sleep wherever and whenever the opportunity presents itself.

Not everybody will wish to avail themselves of strategies such as the use of melatonin, artificial light, hypnotic drugs or stimulants. This chapter therefore includes many 'natural' ways of expediting sleeping or staying awake.

Let's look at a typical example:

You are sitting at your desk in London at 9 a.m. on a Wednesday morning when you are suddenly ordered to go to Los Angeles that afternoon. A number of flights are available but let us say you take the BA283, departing London Heathrow at 1200 hrs and arriving in LA at 1500 hrs local time. You are therefore arriving in the middle of the afternoon, quite likely to bright sunshine, when in fact your body clock is telling you that it is 11 p.m. at night (an eight-hour time difference).

You are faced therefore with a choice. Do you give in to your body clock and collapse straight into bed but run the risk of waking up spontaneously at one o'clock in the morning? Or do you attempt to stay awake for another eight hours in the knowledge that if you can manage this you will almost certainly fall asleep until the following morning and will be on LA time when you wake up?

In another scenario you may be sitting in your office in New York and be suddenly requested to depart for London. You catch the 'red eye' with whatever airline suits you and arrive in Heathrow at 0600 hrs. You have had 5–6 hours of fitful sleep and your own clock is telling you it is 1100 hrs and you should be at work. You either stay awake and get on with it, or you risk having a few hours sleep – but what will you feel like when you wake up, *if* you wake up?! Clearly, here, the better strategy is to stay awake even though you might feel tired.

So, having decided whether to adopt the staying-awake or going-to-sleep tactic, how can you help yourself to implement these approaches? Let us now examine the many variables that you can use to this end.

Exercise

Virtually every five-star hotel is equipped with either a gym or a swimming pool or both. A gym kit in your travel bag is strongly recommended. It need not be elaborate. All that is required is shorts, a tee shirt and sensible underclothes. Running shoes are not necessary. Boxer shorts can double as swimming trunks. Quite apart from the health benefits to be gained from such exercise it is actually quite difficult to fall asleep immediately following vigorous exercise, so it can be used as a staying-awake tactic. It is more difficult to go to sleep at night following a bout of stiff exercise than without.[68]

Even if you are a person who does not wish to engage in formal exercise as such, almost any other brisk activity will suffice. Go for a walk, or do some stretching exercises. Some people find that even chewing gum helps them to stay alert, but *do not do this in Singapore*, where it is illegal!

Half an hour of exercise will keep you alert for up to two hours afterwards.[69] Many people who jog will notice that if they do so last thing at night, sleep is often quite difficult to come by.

Being stuck in an aircraft is no excuse for not exercising. It is perfectly possible to take exercise without ever leaving your seat. Many airlines describe such exercises in their in-flight magazines. Some airlines even have the cabin crew run through the exercises with the passengers before landing, to help you loosen up. You can do these exercises if you need to stay awake when you land.

Environmental temperature and humidity

There are two extremes to this spectrum. On the one hand, cold dry air helps to maintain alertness, while a warm humid background is soporific. Alertness is therefore enhanced in a cold climate by throwing the windows open, and in the Far East (say) by turning up the air-conditioning.

Similarly, a warm shower turning then to cold will freshen you up, whereas a hot bath will bring on a desire to sleep.

People seem to sleep better when the surrounding temperature is closest to their 'thermal comfort zone'. This is that narrow band of temperature where it is neither so cold that you have to increase your metabolic rate or shiver to stay warm, nor so hot that you have to sweat to keep cool. The average temperature of the 'thermal comfort zone' is about 25°C (77°F) though there is some variation according to body size.[70] If you want to sleep, make sure the surrounding temperature is at or about this level. Conversely, if you wish to stay awake, turn the heating or air-conditioning up or down so as to get away from these 'comfort' temperatures.

If you have access to an ionizer, it is claimed that negative ions can maintain alertness. In addition there is some evidence that an ionizer improves the quality of sleep when used at night, especially if you suffer from allergies.[71]

Environmental background light

Bright light stimulates alertness whereas dim light encourages a feeling of relaxation and ultimately sleep. You cannot always control ambient light but it is generally easier to make things dimmer, e.g., by wearing sunglasses. If you need more brightness in your hotel room, turn all the lights on. After all, you or your company are paying for it so you are entitled to use the electricity. Some travellers bring their own portable source of light. A photographic lamp with a 500 or 1000 watt bulb is ideal, or you can walk around with your own headset of inbuilt light (see Chapter 10).

Onboard, if you require bright daylight and the shutters are down to show the movie, just explain the situation and the hostess will accommodate you in alternative seating.

Psychological stimuli

If you occupy your time and engage yourself in activity where you yourself are required to provide an input, this will obviously keep you awake more than lying back and remaining passive. When reading a newspaper, for example, to remain awake it is better to do the crossword or solve the chess problem than just to read the text.

Go over your presentation, get worked up about it, worry about the questions that might be asked of you. Work on your laptop.

Take a walk downtown, crossing streets, avoiding traffic and keeping an eye out for muggers or pickpockets. All of this will raise your alertness. Take your shopping list with you and use this 'dead time' to fill the orders. The following day you can then use your free time to enjoy yourself instead of doing chores.

Environmental sound

Bring your walkman. Avoid baroque (Bach, Vivaldi, etc) and Mozart – all excellent composers, but likely to send one to sleep! Far better to bring selections of loud rock or pop music. The radio side of your walkman won't work on board but once you arrive try to find a station broadcasting in English, or in your own language. A chat show, particularly if there is interaction between various people expressing differing opinions, will stimulate you to stay awake more than any music can.

Sleep bank

Laboratory experiments have demonstrated that reducing a night's sleep impairs alertness the following day.[72] So if you normally need eight hours sleep per night, make sure that you do get this amount for the few days preceding your departure. It is easy not to, particularly if you are an infrequent traveller and get nervous at the prospect of flying.

Comfort

The more comfortable one's surroundings, the easier it is to fall asleep. The converse is equally true, hence the old story about someone's propensity for a nap being so great that they 'could sleep on a clothes line'.

The quality of the comfort in aircraft accommodation obviously varies with cabin class. Economy can be pretty uncomfortable, particularly on charter flights, whereas the comforts of First Class can almost equate to those of home. Travelling First or Business class therefore works in your favour if you are trying to get some sleep on the plane but against you if you are trying to stay awake. In any case, when trying to stay awake, pick an aisle seat so that you can take frequent walks up and down the aircraft.

The same goes for posture. EEG recordings (recordings of brain electrical activity) tell us that people sleeping in comfortable armchairs do not get good-quality sleep. The amount of so-called slow-wave sleep (the deepest) is virtually nil, and they spend most of the night hovering between the two lightest stages of sleep.[73] The message is clear: to stay awake, stay vertical. To get quality sleep you must lie as horizontally as possible.

If you are trying to stay awake in your hotel room, do

not lounge on the bed watching TV. Sitting upright and in a slightly uncomfortable chair is better.

When out and about, a small stone in your shoe will work wonders. The discomfort produced will certainly help to keep you awake. And always remember that the enemy of alertness is monotony.

Food and drink

There are many common foods and drinks which, apart from their ability to nourish us, are capable of making us more alert (stimulants) or calmer and sleepier (depressants). The commonest stimulant is caffeine, which we all know is present in coffee. Appreciable amounts are also found in tea, more particularly if the tea has 'stewed' by the time it gets to you (a common occurrence on airlines).

Chocolate is another stimulant, containing not only caffeine but another wake-you-up drug called Theobromine along with traces of other chemicals related to amphetamine. The darker the chocolate, the greater the stimulant effect.

Late-night drinks such as hot chocolate and cocoa also contain enough caffeine to disturb sleep. Many soft drinks also contain caffeine. These can include Coca Cola, Pepsi Cola, Dr. Pepper, Mountain Dew and Sunkist Orange. Check the packaging to see if a particular drink does contain caffeine, and if so, how much.

Sleepiness and alertness are closely related to the amount of a chemical called serotonin that happens to be in the brain at any one time. The more there is, the sleepier you are. Serotonin is made from an amino acid called tryptophan. Research carried out in the Massachusetts Institute of Technology has shown that eating something rich in tryptophan raises the level of serotonin in the brain. There are two ways to accomplish this: the direct and the indirect. Rich sources of tryptophan include milk, yoghurt and ice cream, chicken, turkey and tuna.

The indirect way is to eat carbohydrates (foods containing sugar). Through a complex mechanism involving insulin, this raises the amount of tryptophan in the blood (from body stores). Both of these tricks will work better if taken with Vitamin B6.[74]

Proprietary medicines

A large number of over-the-counter medicines for common minor conditions such as coughs and colds, or hay fever, contain drugs some of which are stimulant and others depressant. The stimulant ones will help you to stay awake, and the depressant ones will help you to sleep (but they will not make you depressed!). The problem lies in not being aware of their effects. You could, for example, be lying in bed having taken some Pseudoephedrine for a blocked up nose, and wondering why you can't get to sleep!

The following table lists a number of such drugs according to their stimulant or depressant properties.

STIMULANTS	DEPRESSANTS
Ephedrine	Brompheniramine
Phenylephrine	Carbinoxamine
Phenylpropanolamine	Chlorpheniramine
Pseudoephedrine	Diphenhydramine
Theophylline	Doxylamine
Xylometazoline	Pheniramine
	Phenyltoloxamine
	Promethazine
	Triprolidine

A little known but very useful property of common aspirin is that it helps to keep you asleep once you get there. Research carried out in the Mayo Clinic has shown that two aspirin at bedtime decreases the number of night-time awakenings and increases the total time spent asleep. Its effect is mostly in the latter half of the night, so it is particularly helpful for those who can get off to sleep but have trouble staying there.

Knowing now the properties of these common drugs, you can use them yourself as an aid to sleeping or staying awake as you see fit. But do read the manufacturer's label before taking any drug.

Stimulants

We mentioned above the stimulant effect of caffeine found in food and drinks, but of course caffeine itself can be bought in pure tablet form from chemists' shops.

Amphetamines such as Dexamphetamine have been out of favour with the medical profession for some decades as a result of their potential for addiction when taken carelessly. They do, however, have a long and respectable history. As well as being one of the earliest drugs to treat depression successfully, in World War II they were given to British pilots to sustain them during long and repeated bombing missions.

More recently, amphetamines have been used by American troops (supplied by their physicians!) in the conflicts in the Middle East. Dextroamphetamine (5 mg every four hours) was used effectively and without major side effects in tactical flying operations during operations Desert Storm and Desert Shield in Iraq.[75] It should be noted, though, that this was approved only for pilots who had been given the drug on the ground, and were side-effect free, and were subject to close flight-surgeon supervision.

This author is not for a moment suggesting that you should fly off into the sunset with a handful of Dexedrine in your pocket to 'give it a go'. However, if the USAF is prepared to allow multi-million dollar aircraft, such as the A-10 Thunderbolt 11 and the F–16 Fighting Falcon, to be flown by pilots with these drugs inside them, there may just be something in the idea.

Alcohol

Alcohol is an important sedative which can usefully be employed as a 'sleeping pill'. In view of the additional historical and social aspects of alcohol, and the importance of using it wisely, a fuller discussion of its role and effects is given later in Chapter 13.

Herbal and homeopathic remedies

There is a wide range of these, and again they have the advantage of having been around for so long that much is known about their potential toxic effects. Amongst the more successful for inducing sleep are passionflower, camomile, valerian root, lettuce tea, hops and pulsatilla. But these are not easily found everywhere in the world and when they can be found their purity or strength may be very variable. The traveller relying on these will therefore almost certainly have to bring his or her own supply.

Hypnotism

Many people have learnt auto-hypnotism: the ability to hypnotize oneself into (amongst other things) going off to sleep at will. This is particularly helpful for those who eschew sleeping pills, alcohol and herbal remedies. In the UK, commercial hypnotists are listed in the Yellow

Pages, and the British Society of Medical and Dental Hypnosis can provide you with a list of doctors or dentists in your area who can teach you to hypnotize yourself. (See Appendix A for contact details.)

Sleeping pills

There is a very wide variety of sleeping pills on the market, available by doctor's prescription. They all have differing properties in terms of their speed of onset, duration of action, propensity to produce hangover, and indeed their suitability at all if you suffer from any disease.

A list of commonly available sleeping pills and their various properties can be found in Appendix C.

The longer a sleeping pill stays in your bloodstream, the more likely overall it is to produce a hangover effect.[76]

Picking the right sleeping pill is important. Suppose for example you arrive at your destination at 0430 hrs and your hotel is right next-door to the airport. You could be in bed by 0500 hrs and would like to get 4–5 hours of sleep before your first meeting at midday. Being an owl, you are quite happy to get up at 1000 hrs but find it difficult to get off to sleep in a strange hotel. Zolpidem or Zopiclone would be good for you under these circumstances. They each have a rapid onset of action, last 4–6 hours and have minimal hangover effect.

But now suppose you arrive in Los Angeles from London at 1515 hrs local time. You have decided to adopt the sleeping strategy, so need something to keep you asleep for a good 16 hours. A good choice here would be Nitrazepam/Mogodon as this is a long-acting drug.

The precise effect of any sleeping pill on an individual can be quite variable, so you are well advised to first try out at home whatever you intend to use abroad.

You are now armed with a good number of potential tactics to help you to either stay awake or go to sleep on demand. There should be enough choice here to suit everyone's tastes. A summary of these tactics appears in Appendix B.

9

Melatonin

As was explained in Chapter 1, when we are awake virtually no melatonin is produced by the pineal gland and conversely it is during the hours of darkness, while we sleep, that we produce all our melatonin.

It therefore follows that it might be possible to use melatonin to regulate the day/night cycle, and indeed this turns out to be the case.

In the first place melatonin can be used to induce sleep. It has been shown that a small dose of melatonin can induce sleep in healthy volunteers – i.e., people who have no difficulty getting to sleep anyway.[77] It can also get you off to sleep faster.[78]

Furthermore it has been shown that elderly patients with chronic insomnia have low production levels of melatonin at night and that, taken at bedtime, melatonin can restore to normality the poor sleep pattern of these patients.[79]

But can melatonin help with jetlag?

The answer is a resounding YES.

As far back as ten years ago, Prof. J. Arendt and her team from the University of Surrey flew 17 volunteers from London to San Francisco, where they remained for two weeks before being flown back again. The results were staggering, there being an enormous difference in the time that it took to recover from jetlag between those who took supplementary melatonin and those who took a placebo, even though neither the volunteers nor the doctors measuring the jetlag knew who was taking which.[80]

These results were confirmed three years later by Keith Petrie and his team from New Zealand, who did a field study of 20 volunteers on flights between Auckland and London and back and found the same amazing results.[81]

The bottom line is that melatonin reduces the time it takes to adjust to any given new time zone. It acts as a sort of overrider switch, tuning you in to your destination. The power of melatonin to effect this has become legend amongst the travelling classes, and justifiably so.

But how exactly do you make melatonin work for you?

The secret, as with so many things in life, is in the timing.

You use melatonin as an ON switch: to induce not only sleep but also all the biological changes associated with sleep. The best way to demonstrate this is by some examples.

Let's say you are taking the London/Singapore flight and you have decided to travel with Air Singapore on SQ319, departing London Heathrow at 1100 hrs and arriving at Changi at 0745 hrs the following morning. As you are going for a week you cannot use the In&Out strategy and so will have to adjust your own clock to Singapore time as quickly as possible. So you correctly decide to set your own clock to Singapore time before you depart. This happens to be eight hours ahead of Britain at the time of your trip. It is therefore 1900 hrs in Singapore when you leave London, so you correctly stay awake for the first 4–5 hours of the flight to have a cocktail, dinner, perhaps watch the movie, and then turn in for the night. But when you are attempting to go off to sleep your own body clock will be on about 3 o'clock in the afternoon – not the easiest thing to do without help.

So you take your melatonin at this time, together with either your chosen sleeping pill or alcoholic nightcap. You sleep for 7–8 hours and wake up, in time for pre-landing, to a Singapore morning. Hopefully you will then be set for a full day's work before retiring to bed, pleasantly tired, at about 11 p.m. Singapore time. At this time your body will still be a little confused. The zeitgebers are telling you it is indeed bedtime but the inbuilt clock is still holding on to the idea that it is only three o'clock in the afternoon, and so will still show some signs of reluctance to allow you to nod off. You can, however, persuade it that it really is 11 p.m. after all by taking melatonin at this time. And you should continue to take your melatonin at this time for the first 4–5 nights. This is to prevent your body clock slipping back into London time.

On the return journey things are reversed. You avoid the SQ320 as this departs Changi at 1230 local time. This equates to 0430 hrs in London, when you should be asleep. Instead the wise traveller will take the SQ322, departing at 2315 hrs from Changi and arriving at Heathrow at 0530 hrs. On departure it is 3.15 in the afternoon in London, so you stay awake for say the first eight hours of the flight: using, if necessary, a light box. You then take your melatonin with or without sleeping pill or nightcap, as above. This should allow you to get the best part of six hours sleep and, on your arrival in London, allow you to face a day's work. There will be a temptation to drop off at about 3–4 o'clock in the afternoon, this being 11–12 at night Singapore time. This temptation must be firmly resisted. Come 11 p.m. in London you will paradoxically find that it is now difficult to get off to sleep; not surprisingly, though, as your body clock tells you it is 0700 hours and time to wake up – no matter how tired you feel. In this situation, taking melatonin and the judicious use of alcohol or sleeping pills for a night or two will pay dividends.

Let's now consider a different example so that you can fully familiarize yourself with how melatonin works.

You live in San Francisco and you are going to take your honeymoon in Australia, flying to Sydney.

You decide to take United Airlines flight UA863, departing San Francisco at 2220 hrs and landing in Sydney at 0745. On your departure there is a six-hour time difference. You would normally be settling down for the night at home, but remember it is only 1620 hrs in Sydney. You therefore stay awake for the first 7 hours and 40 minutes hours of this flight (i.e., up to midnight, Sydney time), taking your melatonin and sleeping for as much of the remainder of the flight as the flight attendants will let you. It may not be much fun spending the first night of your honeymoon in an aircraft seat, but that's the sort of price we all have to pay for long-distance travel. (You could have gone to Sacramento and got there before midnight!)

Arriving in Sydney in the early morning, you spend the rest of the day awake and up and about. Then take the melatonin at about 11 p.m., local time, and retire for the night. Carry on with the melatonin for a few nights until you have fully adjusted to Sydney time.

Your honeymoon enjoyably completed, you and your spouse then return on United Airlines flight UA862, which departs Sydney at about 1150 hrs, or 5.50 p.m.

San Francisco time. You again spend the first six hours awake. Your body clock will tell you it is only 5 p.m. yet you are now trying to get off to sleep. A little help is needed, so again you take your melatonin together with whatever else you need, and sleep for the remainder of the flight. You should then arrive in San Francisco at 0710 hrs ready to face a full day, having had a good 6–7 hours sleep. Again you should take the melatonin for a few nights following your return, until your clock is fully back into Californian time.

How safe is taking melatonin?

The answer is: probably extremely safe.

For a start, we all produce it. It is therefore something intrinsic to us – unlike drugs, which are foreign substances. Any seventy-year-old person will have been exposed to melatonin for 70 years without any apparent ill effects. Even subjects exposed to high doses (80mg) displayed increased tiredness only for a few hours and no other ill effects.[82] In one experiment researchers tried to assassinate mice by poisoning them with melatonin. They gave them doses of up to 800mg/kg (equivalent to about 56000mgs in humans) and yet failed to kill a single mouse.[83] In human experiments it was found necessary to administer 3000–6000mgs a day for a month before any side effects were reported, and even these consisted only of abdominal cramps.[84] The only slight reservations I have about the safety of melatonin concerns taking it if you suffer from any of the 'auto-immune' diseases. These are diseases which result when the natural immune system in your body becomes over-exuberant and starts to destroy your own tissues, in the mistaken 'belief' that it is doing its designated job of destroying invading bugs such as viruses and bacteria. Multiple sclerosis, which is thought to be an autoimmune disease, is made worse by melatonin.[85] There is also some evidence that autoimmune arthritis is made worse by melatonin.[86] While these doubts remain, I do not believe that anybody suffering from an autoimmune disease should take melatonin supplements. A table listing autoimmune diseases can be found in Appendix D at the back of this book. If you are in any doubts as to whether you suffer from one of these illnesses, you should check with your doctor. Fortunately, with the exception of rheumatoid arthritis, the autoimmune diseases are not common.

For those travellers not affected by autoimmune diseases, how much melatonin should be taken?

Most of the research done has reported success with 5mgs,[87,88,89] with one study recommending 8mgs.[90]

Melatonin usually comes in capsules containing either 2.5 or 3mgs. It can be stored at room temperature until the expiry date, is rapidly and almost completely absorbed by mouth,[91] and its effect lasts for about one to two hours. There is some person-to-person variation, so if a dose of 5mgs does not produce the desired effect within an hour it is worthwhile experimenting with up to 20mgs. Even taking a dosage of 75mgs of melatonin improves alertness the following day in poor sleepers.[92]

In the USA melatonin is regarded as a food supplement and so does not come under the regulatory auspices of the Food and Drug Administration (FDA). It can therefore be legally bought and sold in health-food shops.

In Great Britain the situation is different. An expert committee of the Medicines Control Agency (or MCA, the British equivalent of the American FDA) has decided that melatonin cannot be regarded as a foodstuff and therefore is subject to the same regulations that govern the marketing of a drug. In Britain nobody can advertise or sell a drug to the public without such a drug having a product licence. Obtaining a product licence is a difficult and expensive procedure, with much research having to be submitted to the MCA. Once a product licence is granted it applies to the drug and not the applicant, so unless your drug is protected by a patent (and melatonin has no patent, being a natural substance and relatively easy to manufacture) anybody can make use of that licence to sell the said product to the public. There is therefore no incentive for anybody to apply for such a product licence, and so a sort of Catch 22 situation applies.

Fortunately the UK has some doctors who understand the benefits as well as the risk of using melatonin and are happy to prescribe and dispense it to suitable patients. Page 119 explains how to get in touch with one of these doctors.

As regards the future, a great deal of work still needs to be done to determine how effective melatonin is in rapidly shifting the myriad physiological functions in the body to a new time zone, and indeed to find the most effective dose to achieve this.

Meanwhile, as Prof. R.V. Short, Professor of reproductive biology at Monash University (Victoria, Australia), puts it:

'The evidence that taking melatonin benefits jetlagged travellers . . . becomes stronger by the day.'[93]

Light

Just as we can use melatonin to induce sleep and put the body on 'night mode', so we can also use bright light to put our bodies on 'day mode'. This can then accelerate the adaptive changes our body clocks have to make when travelling across time zones.

Just as melatonin is produced by our pineal glands during the hours of darkness conversely no melatonin is produced by day, with the exception of a small surge after lunch. Ever wonder why you feel a little sleepy after lunch? This has become enshrined in the custom of the siesta in Mediterranean countries.

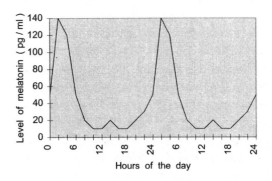

So what happens if we are exposed to light at night-time. It all depends on the strength of the light. Light intensity is measured in a unit called a *lux* (which is Latin for light). As a rough approximation, 500 lux is about the strength of background light at home or in industrial conditions in the evening with electric lighting being used – i.e., bright enough to see exactly what you are doing. 2500 lux, by contrast, is about the intensity of light you would experience from indirect sunlight when standing by a window on a clear spring day. Whereas a dose of 500 lux has little or no effect, on suppressing melatonin, 700–800 lux begins to do so. 1000 lux does the job adequately, and maximum suppression (no melatonin production) occurs at exposures of 2000–2500 lux.

Furthermore it is known that bright light can actually alter human circadian rhythms, and this is thought to occur by the same process of melatonin suppression.[94] A number of experiments have established light therapy as an effective method of altering the body clock.[95,96,97]

Light therapy therefore offers a method of altering the body clock for those who would rather avoid hormones, drugs or alcohol, and would prefer instead to use a natural method of control. It should of course be used alongside the strategy of picking the best available flights.

With light therapy, generally, you are embarking on trips where the objective is to stay awake against your natural inclination. The use of light facilitates this by suppressing your melatonin production. The therapy should therefore be used alongside the staying-awake strategies described in Chapter 7. It is important to note that light therapy can be employed successfully both in the air and on the ground.

To be effective, the source must be capable of exposing your eyeballs to at least 800 lux of light. The physics of this is quite complex and in any case need not trouble the layman. It will suffice to note here that the strength of light diminishes by the square of the distance from its source. Thus, if you have a light which is delivering to you 2000 lux when you are at a distance of one metre from it, the same light will only deliver 500 lux when you are two metres away from it. (2 squared is 4, and 2000 divided by 4 is 500.)

There are basically two ways of producing this sort of light. The first is to use purpose-built portable light visors such as those made by Bio-Brite Inc. These devices deliver between 800 and 3000 lux of adjustable light to you and are comfortable to wear. As explained earlier, 2000 lux is more than adequate and I feel there is nothing to be gained by setting this equipment to its maximum setting of 3000 lux.

Alternatively, you can bring a plug-in source of light to use in your hotel room, or wherever. The easiest such source is a photographic light bulb of 500 or 1000 watts. With one of these plugged in, you can walk around your hotel room and still be exposed to enough lux to favourably alter your rhythms.

As with taking supplementary melatonin, with light therapy timing is vital. This is illustrated by the following examples.

You are flying home to LA after an exhibition week in London, so your clock is now firmly on London time. You decide to take American Airlines flight AA137, departing London Heathrow at 1105 hrs and arriving at LA at 1445 hrs local time. On touchdown your body clock is telling you that it is 2245 hrs and hence that you are due for a good sleep fairly shortly. However, if you are to facilitate your speedy return to LA time you must stay awake for another eight hours or so. This is where the light therapy comes into its own. If you expose yourself to at least 2000 lux for seven hours this will do the trick and you should repeat this for a further few days until you feel firmly back on LA time. In summer, of course, the first 2–3 hours will be provided by the sun itself if you stay out of doors.

Now suppose you are off on a business trip to Kuala Lumpur, in Malaysia, from your base in London. You have been booked on flight MH1 with Malaysian Airlines. This flight departs London Heathrow at 2200 hrs, which, for reasons explained above, is not at all ideal. (I.e., you are up and about when everyone in KL is asleep.) Flight MH 3, departing from London at 1050 hrs, would be preferable, but let us assume that the MH1 flight has been prebooked for you and that you are stuck with it. Keen to compensate for someone else's bad choice, you now wish to adjust to Malaysian time as quickly as possible. Being eight hours ahead, the time in Kuala Lumpur is 0600 hrs when you leave Heathrow. So the best you can hope for is about two hours sleep. You will then have to stay awake for the remaining ten hours of the flight. It is of course (being winter) pitch black outside for the first six hours, until you are over the Middle East and dawn is approaching. So the trick is to have a nap for the first couple of hours on this flight. Then wear your light visor for the next few hours until it becomes sufficiently bright outside. Eight hours after departure there will be enough light by the starboard window seats to dispense with the visor. (Starboard is defined as the right-hand side when you are facing the front of the plane.)

The evidence suggests that light therapy is completely safe. Because of the wavelengths being used (the visible spectrum, with no ultra-violet component) there is no risk of developing skin cancer from being exposed to bright light for hours on end. Common sense, however, dictates that it would be foolish to stare directly at a 1000-watt light bulb for any length of time.

In summary, light therapy offers a safe and effective method of combating jetlag, and the technology now exists to deliver this promise.

11

Sleep Deprivation

Of course when you are using light to stay awake, when you would otherwise be asleep, you can expect to experience the ill effects of sleep deprivation. These ill effects share some of the characteristics of jetlag, such as inappropriate sleepiness,[98] and in addition they worsen the decline in performance that is associated with jetlag.

It is very important to catch up on this sleep deficit if performance is to be restored. An example shows how this is achieved.

Imagine for a moment that you get on a plane in London and fly to Tokyo, change and fly then to Los Angeles. You change again and finally arrive back in London. You have ignored my advice in Chapter 6 and are travelling eastward. You could do this trip using a combination of British Airways, Singapore Airlines and Japanese Airlines, and your total flying time would be about 35 hours. Allowing say 13 hours for changing planes, let's say that you should arrive back in London 48 hours after you left. Because you were back in your original time zone within two days you would experience relatively little jetlag (compared with staying in each city for 24 hours or more). However, because, for one reason or another, you have stayed awake for the entire two days, you would now have a very serious sleep deficit and would be feeling a complete wreck!

If you would normally sleep eight hours per night,

you now have a deficit of 16 hours. The symptoms of sleep depravation are, I'm sure, familiar to all of us. Apart from an at-times overwhelming desire to sleep there is increased irritability and a sharp decline in our intellectual abilities. Numerous experiments have shown that there is a sharp and serious decline in our alertness, concentration and memory, resulting from sleep deprivation, even though we may not be aware of it at the time.[99,100]

The nuclear fallout at Chernobyl, the oil spillage from the 'Exxon Valdez', the near meltdown at Three Mile Island and the loss of the space shuttle Challenger, were all caused by the same thing. People made mistakes with disastrous consequences because they were trying to make decisions when they had had insufficient sleep.[101] If you think you couldn't screw up your company's business in the same way . . . dream on! (It is possible to test yourself to see if sleep deprivation has resulted in a temporary decline in your intellectual abilities. Kits for doing this are available from the Jetlag Clinic. See page 119.)

If we have to perform in a sleep-deprived state, there is usually a surge in wellbeing together with an improvement in our alertness and concentration between about 7–9 a.m. and again around 7–9 p.m. Do not be fooled, however: these peaks are followed by quite severe troughs when we are fairly worthless from a work-capacity point of view.

It is therefore essential to restore any sleep deficit. Obviously if you go to bed and sleep off the whole 16 hours you will create a jetlag-type situation in exactly the same way as a shift worker would – so you are no better off doing that. The trick is to build the catching-up into your normal sleeping pattern. If you are a lark, go to bed an hour or two earlier. If an owl, sleep on in the morning for an extra hour or two – until the deficit has been restored.

That was a rather extreme example, since, fortunately, most of us never have to go screaming around the world in 48 hours.

Let's look at some examples to illustrate this point. There is a time difference of eight hours between London and Los Angeles. So when you arrive in L.A. after flying from London, your journey westward will produce an elongation of eight hours. Let us say that you normally go to bed at 11 p.m. You went to bed on say Tuesday night at 11 p.m. in London. You therefore want to go to bed at 11 p.m. on Wednesday night in LA. Because of the eight-hour time difference there is an interval of 32 hours (24+8) between bedtime in one country and the next.

Because of your sleep requirements (eight hours for every 24-hour period) you now require an extra one third of eight hours, or two hours and 40 minutes, to catch up.

If you normally need seven hours sleep, the deficit you have to catch up is 2 hours and 20 minutes of sleep (one third of seven), and so on.

Now let's look at the unfortunate businessman who has to get from New York to Bangkok as quickly as possible – a time difference of some 12 hours. He could travel eastward via London or Amsterdam but is sensible enough to follow my advice and fly west via Los Angeles. Flying with American Airlines and Thai Airways International, he can leave home on Monday morning and be in Bangkok by Monday night. Let us say that he needs seven hours sleep every night and that he normally goes to bed at midnight. Having gone to bed at midnight in New York on Sunday night, with the above routing and airlines he can be in bed at midnight in Bangkok. However, there will be an interval of 36 hours between bedtime in New York and bedtime in Bangkok (24 hours plus 12 hours time difference). He will therefore need 10.5 (seven plus half of seven) hours sleep to catch up.

Failure to catch up on this sleep deficit will produce problems additional to those of jetlag in itself.

The problem of sleep deprivation does not arise when flying east, as you are then shortening the day and so, if anything, decreasing the amount of time you need sleep. However, as previously explained, travelling east is liable to produce far worse jetlag than flying west.

12

Women and Jetlag

Women encounter their own unique health problems, some of which can impact on flying and jetlag.

For example, should women subject themselves to repeated jetlag during pregnancy? Unfortunately, very little hard evidence exists to answer this question one way or the other.

A woman who is pregnant is more vulnerable psychologically than at any other stage in her life except the menopause.[102] This vulnerability is due to changes in various hormone levels and indeed men would be just as vulnerable were there some equivalent process they could go through which had such a profound effect on their hormones. It is known that jetlag predisposes susceptible people to adverse emotional and psychological changes. Travelling west is more likely to precipitate depression[103] and is of course more likely to do so in the immediate few weeks following childbirth, when a woman faces the hazards of puerperal depression.[104]

Most airlines permit their air hostesses to work for the first three months of pregnancy. It is during this time that all the important organs are formed in the baby and exposure to flying or to jetlag does not seem to produce any adverse effects on the baby.[105] Certainly if it did produce ill effects, I would have expected airlines to ground these staff members as soon as they knew or suspected they might be pregnant.

Throughout this book various pieces of advice are offered to the traveller about the use of alcohol and various drugs. Whereas a heavy alcohol intake during a pregnancy is harmful both to mother and baby, most doctors would agree that there is no harm in an occasional glass or two of wine. With regard to drugs, in general they should be avoided during pregnancy,[106] especially during the first three months.[107] Some drugs mentioned, such as amphetamine, should never be used during pregnancy.[108] I also advise that the newer sleeping pills, such as Zolpidem and Zopiclone, should not be used, as their manufacturers have yet to establish the safety of their use during pregnancy.[109, 110]

If a sleeping pill is necessary, then an older antihistamine drug is preferable, as these have been around for a long time and any propensity to harm would be more likely to have been detected.[111, 112, 113]

As regards herbal teas and homeopathic remedies, the fact that they are natural products does not in any way guarantee their safety. In fact some herbs have been used historically as abortifacients, i.e., used to cause miscarriage.

It is difficult to make hard and fast rules and I believe women should make up their own minds once they have been given the facts.

An authoritative source takes the view that a woman should not fly in the last third of pregnancy if she is carrying more than one baby, or if there has been any vaginal bleeding prior to flying, or if she has had a premature delivery in the past.[114] I think this is probably sound advice but every case should be decided on its merits. Most airlines will allow pregnant passengers on flights up to the end of their thirty-fourth week of pregnancy.

Repeated long-distance flying of a type likely to produce jetlag has an adverse effect on periods.[115] They become more irregular and when they do occur are more likely to be heavier and/or more painful.[116] This increased irregularity is more likely to result in unplanned pregnancy if rhythm methods of contraception are employed. It also means that premenstrual syndrome is likely to be worse.[117] Many women experience premenstrual fluid retention, resulting in – amongst other effects – swollen ankles. For reasons explained in Chapter 5, there is a drop in cabin pressure shortly after the doors are closed. This will make swollen ankles worse. There is a real danger that if shoes are removed during the flight, for comfort's sake, then you may not be able to get them back on again! My advice is to wear looser-fitting shoes and to keep them on during the flight.

Taking the combined oral contraceptive (the type that contains oestrogen and a progestogen) increases the chances of getting a blood clot in the legs.[118] Furthermore, the immobility produced by sitting for a long period, together with the dehydrating effect of flying, makes this risk even greater. Indeed, this risk has been labelled 'economy leg syndrome', in recognition of the part that immobility plays in its genesis.[119] The woman traveller taking the oral contraceptive needs therefore to be aware of this risk, and should take adequate precautions, including adequate fluid intake and in-flight exercise, to minimize the risk.

Women who take the progestogen-only pill are told, or should be told, that it is important to take it at the same time each day.[120] Forgetting to take the pill for one day, or even just taking it a few hours late, can have disastrous consequences. You are unlikely to encounter problems when staying put in the same place. But what happens when you travel large distances rapidly?

There is no problem when flying east, as you are shortening the day and therefore if anything taking more than you need. However, when you travel west you elongate the day and can therefore be stretching out the distance between doses. Let's say you are based in London and are on a progestogen-only (or mini) pill. Let's say you always take it at about eight o clock in the morning. You get an invitation to go to Hollywood for the Oscars! So you jump on a plane and fly to Los Angeles. However, if you wait until eight o'clock the following morning in Los Angeles to take your next pill, the interval between pills will be 32 hours. (A full day plus the eight-hour time difference.) This delay can be critical with this particular type of contraceptive. You should instead take your next pill at midnight when you arrive, as this equates to eight o'clock the following morning in London. You would then continue to take it at midnight every night as long as you remain in Los Angeles, and switch back to the eight in the morning timing when you arrive back in London.

When travelling abroad, always take a supply of anti-diarrhoeal tablets with you. These can be prescription-only tablets such as Lomotil, or over-the-counter medications such as Immodium. The importance of having these to hand is as follows. Although, apart from the inconvenience, diarrhoea in itself does not do you great harm, nevertheless even with a moderately severe attack you are passing out at the other end the contraceptive pill that you swallowed only a couple of hours ago. You therefore need to bear in mind that unless you bring the diarrhoea under control pretty quickly you will be losing all contraceptive protective cover. On a honeymoon you could therefore be starting a family rather sooner than you might have planned!

Always, always carry your contraceptive pills and indeed any other medication that you have to take on a regular basis in your hand luggage. You might think you know when you are going to land but delays do occur and of course they are unpredictable.

Worse, your checked baggage can go missing. If you lose your pills it can often be tricky as well as expensive to get replacements in a foreign country. Quite often with the combined oral contraceptive pill you cannot get the exact equivalent abroad. If you therefore switch to a different variety you can lay yourself open to new side effects when you least want them – away from home, and upsetting your holiday.

For anatomical reasons, women are far more likely to be afflicted by cystitis than men. Moreover, becoming dehydrated increases the risk of developing this unpleasant condition.[121] As explained in Chapter 5 it is very easy to become dehydrated whilst flying. It is particularly important therefore for women prone to this condition to know that they are more likely to get it when flying unless particular attention is paid to getting enough fluid. And let's face it: the only thing worse than getting cystitis is getting it when you are flying and away from home. As a rough guide to knowing whether you are getting enough fluid, you can judge this by the colour of your urine. The more dehydrated you get, the darker it becomes. You should aim to keep it at a pale yellow colour. Unfortunately, it's difficult to judge this in an aircraft, as the urine does not collect in a white ceramic bowl as on land! If in doubt you can pee into one of the paper cups provided by cabin staff. Sounds disgusting? But perhaps not as bad as getting cystitis and having the embarrassment of having to use the loo every ten minutes.

Many women have a problem with dry skin on their hands and faces. This is often the case due to a slight but unrealized allergy to one or more of the contents of cosmetics used, which produces a very very mild eczema on the skin. For reasons explained in Chapter 5, the atmosphere within a jet aircraft becomes very dry indeed within a few hours of takeoff. If you do indeed suffer from dry skin, it is made worse by flying and particularly by long flights, since the air gets drier and drier as the flight progresses. Unfortunately drinking lots of liquids, while good for you generally, will not help your skin. If preparing for flights lasting more than two to three hours, you should take with you plenty of hand cream and face cream. These creams should be of the unperfumed hypoallergenic type. Generous applications to the skin should be repeated every three to four hours, except when sleeping.

And so we see there are a number of health matters specific to women which can be adversely affected by long-distance flying and jetlag, but which can also be anticipated and to a considerable extent alleviated or avoided thanks to prudent planning.

13

Alcohol

Alcohol plays an important part in the management of jetlag. The generally beneficial effects of alcohol on health when taken the right way are undeniable and undisputed. People who drink in moderation generally live longer than people who do not drink.[122]

Continuous exposure to the pressures of constantly changing time zones produces stress. In addition there is the stress of the meetings and presentations which occur on arrival at our destinations. This stress needs to be relieved at the end of the day. Exercise or meditation can be helpful but are not everybody's idea of fun. Relieving stress should be pleasureful.

The judicious use of alcohol is a time-honoured and culturally enshrined way of doing this and indeed many observers feel that it is precisely this relaxing effect of alcohol which promotes good health.

However, care has to be taken that not too much is consumed as this then has an adverse effect on health. People who drink too much die younger than those who do not drink at all.[123]

The amount of alcohol drunk can be measured in so called units. A unit is the quantity contained in a glass of wine (120 cl size, or about 6 glasses to the bottle), a half pint of normal-strength beer or lager, or a single bar measure of spirits (previously one sixth of a gill, now 25 cl).

It is generally acknowledged by the experts in this field that women can safely drink 14–21 units of alcohol per week and men 21–28 units.

There is complete medical agreement that alcohol is a far safer proposition than the use of tranquillizers in relieving ordinary day-to-day stress.

Yet certain considerations need to be taken on board. If you need more than four units an evening on a continuing basis, to relieve the feelings of stress, then you are drinking too much – and, possibly more importantly, you are being exposed to too much stress. Drinking more than this every evening produces a hangover effect the next day. You don't necessarily have to have a headache the morning after to have drunk enough alcohol to materi-ally impair your performance throughout that following day.[124] Impaired performance leads to not being able to keep up with one's workload or not being 'on the ball'. This tends to produce a feeling of inadequacy, which leads to yet more stress, and so more alcohol is needed to combat this in turn. The end result is a spiral dive of increasing stress, producing increasing alcohol dependence, producing more stress. The secret is to recognize an impending problem before it becomes a real problem and do something sensible about it.

Many people suffer from a feeling of background anxiety about life.[125] This is often worse when you are subjected to more pressure, particularly that of jetlag, and being away from home, family, friends and familiarity. Experience leads us to learn that a little drink can do wonders for relieving that anxiety. Indeed, many people use alcohol to relieve the anxiety of meeting new people in a social setting.

If you are subject to this type of anxiety, and come to rely on alcohol to combat it, you can then fall victim to a different type of trouble: so-called rebound anxiety. If you drink a lot of alcohol the night before, and are already subject to anxiety, you are particularly likely to get an attack of severe anxiety the following day between the hours of about midday and 4 p.m.

That can have disastrous consequences if you are in any case fearful of flying and find yourself just about to get on a plane or are stuck on a plane with no alcohol available. It could also sabotage your performance in a crucial meeting.

Do not come to rely on alcohol to relieve anxiety for any length of time. If you do, it will catch up with you. There are specific techniques and drugs that can be used successfully to relieve this problem and a quiet chat with your own doctor can usually help you in the right direction.

Many businessmen are in the habit of drinking quite a lot of alcohol without ever getting drunk. This can easily happen if, for example, lunch each day is preceded by a gin and tonic and accompanied by a half a bottle of wine. Then in the evening another gin and tonic before dinner, half a bottle of wine with dinner, followed by some postprandial brandy or whisky. This particular pattern of drinking – i.e., not bingeing, but continuous – is particularly likely to induce depression in susceptible individuals. In addition, arriving at a destination after a long flight when travelling from a more easterly direction (e.g., arriving in Heathrow from Singapore) is likely to induce a depression in the susceptible.[126]

If while reading this you decide that you are in fact drinking too much, do not under any circumstances stop suddenly, particularly when abroad. It is not difficult to become physically dependant on alcohol. For someone who is dependant in this way, abrupt withdrawal can precipitate a very unpleasant series of changes which, at their worst, culminate in delirium tremens (or the DT's). By all means reduce your daily intake gradually, and seek out expert help as soon as you get back home.

Alcohol is a very useful hypnotic. It can help us to sleep when we might otherwise find it difficult or impossible to sleep. In addition, it has advantages over modern sleeping pills.

Having been used for thousands of years, alcohol's effects on humans is pretty well charted. We are very unlikely to suddenly discover that alcohol can cause this or that previously unrecognized side effect, whereas this is always a risk with drugs – particularly the newer ones.

Alcohol has the further advantages of not requiring a doctor's prescription, being free on aeroplanes, and easily added to your hotel bill!

It also has the advantage of predictability. In other words, you know from experience just how much you need to send you to sleep and how much you can get away with without producing a hangover.

Alcohol also has some disadvantages as a 'sleeping pill'. Though quite good at getting us off to sleep, it is not very good at keeping us there. Analyses of subjects' sleep patterns while under its influence reveal that the quality of the sleep is not very good.

Additionally alcohol is a diuretic, so it makes you want to pass more urine, even when you are asleep. This can wake up the susceptible from a badly wanted night's sleep, and if you are a middle-aged man with an impending prostate problem, the whole business of trying to get a good night's sleep aided by alcohol can be more trouble than it is worth.

The diuretic downside can be minimized by sticking to drinks of higher proof strengths. That way you reduce the volume you drink, and your kidneys have a smaller fluid load to cope with. They just have to deal with the purely diuretic effect of alcohol without the added problem of the fluid load of (say) three pints of lager.

Other large-volume drinks to be avoided as nightcaps are the longer cocktails, such as daiquiris and screwdrivers, and also gin taken with a lot of tonic.

Better is wine, especially red wine, including the more soporific clarets and red riojas. White wine and champagne taken late at night are more likely to wake you up with heartburn or indigestion. Probably best of all are those spirits that can be taken neat, such as whisky, brandy, cognac and some of the liqueurs. Be warned though that too much spirit taken late at night can cause you to awaken a few hours later with unpleasant palpitations.

In summary, alcohol has the capacity to do enormous good but when misused has the capability of causing immense harm. In the battle against jetlag, the fundamental wisdom regarding alcohol is simple but vital. ***Never*** take alcohol when you need to remain alert and sharp. (Consider, perhaps, just how happy you would be to see the pilot with a bottle of vodka!) But when sleepiness does not matter, and especially if it is actively welcome, then a moderate drink or two is not only medically permissible but should be a positive pleasure besides.

14

Practical Flight Management

This chapter puts our theories into practice by detailing jetlag-beating procedures for three very commonly undertaken journeys. It is important to pre-plan just as you would for an important business meeting, and we assume that you will be staying in your destination for more than a few days, and that you will therefore wish to switch your body clock as swiftly and effectively as possible to destination time.

Since flying east is the worst jetlag beast, let's begin with two examples of flights in that direction.

New York ✈ London

This is a very popular flight indeed, with many airlines vying for your custom. Unfortunately this has not necessarily produced the choice of flights that it might have.

There are two basic approaches to this trip, and your choice very much depends on whether you find it easy or difficult to sleep on an aeroplane, and whether you find it easier to sleep or stay awake, on command, the following day. You can treat it as an overnight flight or as a daytime flight. Let's look at the overnight approach first.

The total flying time is only just over seven hours. This creates problems if you are going to use the flight as your night's sleep. Allowing for the time that you are compelled to keep your seat upright during ascent and again during descent, it works out to be a pretty short night's sleep indeed. Nevertheless, the game plan is as follows. Assuming you are going to Great Britain for some time, you will be wise to switch your body clock to British time as quickly as possible and therefore you will start to do this even before you leave. London being five hours ahead of New York, you start doing things five hours ahead. Thus, you have your dinner in New York at around four or five o'clock in the afternoon (as this is nine to ten o'clock in the evening in London).

Enjoy some wine with this meal if it would normally accompany your evening meal.

A suitable flight to pick would be Virgin Atlantic VS4, departing JFK at 1930 hrs. Allow yourself a comfortable period of time to get from your New York restaurant to check in, as having to rush will make it more difficult to get to sleep on the plane. Use the loo and brush your teeth at the airport. Just before boarding – and you need to be sure that you are actually boarding with no delays – you take your melatonin, together with your chosen sleeping pill, or herbal hypnotic, or nightcap. This should all begin to take effect nicely just around the time that you are allowed to recline your seat. You can use eyemasks and earplugs to reduce light and sound if and as necessary. Ideally you should stay asleep until awoken by cabin crew to regain an upright position with your seat, so you should tell them early on in the flight that you do not wish to be awoken for breakfast and should be allowed to sleep until the last possible moment! There is plenty of time to get breakfast in London after landing.

If you are an owl and dislike such an early start to the day you can instead book Virgin Atlantic VS10, which departs JFK at the later time of 2255 hrs, arriving at 1035 hrs in London HRW the following day. You will, however, get an even shorter night's sleep this way, as you should ensure that you awake to have breakfast on the plane at your usual time.

The advent of high-speed travel has not served the traveller well for this particular trip. How much more comfortable it would be if it took two to three hours longer: allowing you to dine at the airport, get a solid eight hours' sleep, enjoy breakfast aboard, and touch down at about 9 a.m.! In any event, it is essential that you stay awake on your first day in London until your normal bedtime. Under no circumstances should you succumb to even a short nap.

Those who find staying awake like that very difficult are better off taking a daytime flight. An example would be United Airlines UA908, departing JFK at 0915 hrs and touching down in London at 2115 hrs. You will have to get out of bed really quite early on the morning of your departure for this take-off time but that is actually good. Say you actually rise at 0500 hrs. This is the equivalent of 1000 hrs in London, which, if anything, would be a bit of a lie-in! So, you have a very early breakfast and then eat your meals for the rest of the day based on London time. You should book a seat on the right-hand or starboard side of the plane, preferably a window one, to maximize the amount of light you are exposed to. You should not nap during the flight and can use the time to get some work done. Eat dinner on board, and the touchdown time of 2100 hrs will get you home or to your hotel just in time for bed. You are very unlikely to need alcohol or a sleeping pill, as so many social cues are there, but you may enjoy a moderate nightcap and you should take your melatonin to help accelerate the clock change.

The following morning you should immediately expose yourself to lots of stimulation; cold shower, bright light, loud radio (spouse permitting!), and so forth. This is to kick-start your clock into realizing that it is daytime. (Remember that if you are getting up at, say, 0730 hrs, your clock will be trying to tell you that it is only 0230 hrs and that you should therefore still be asleep.) After a normal breakfast, you should (having had your requisite eight hours sleep), now be ready to face anything.

Continuing east:

London → Singapore

You are flying at a time of year when Singapore is eight hours ahead of London. A good flight to choose would be British Airways BA11, departing from London HRW at 1100 hrs, lasting 12 hours and 50 minutes, and arriving in Singapore at 0750 hrs the following morning.

To facilitate a rapid change you should wake up as early as possible on the morning of your departure. If this means that you go to bed earlier the night before, in order to get a sufficient number of hours sleep, so much the better.

From the moment you wake up on departure day, you THINK Singapore time – i.e., you do things as if you were eight hours ahead, no matter what cues you are getting from London time. So, for example, if you get up at 0500 hrs London time, you don't have breakfast – you have lunch! Because it is 1 p.m. in Singapore.

Get straight into the normal rush of things that you would be doing in a typical afternoon, even though the rest of the world seems to be just waking up. On boarding the plane at 1100 hrs London time, remember it is now seven o'clock in the evening in Singapore. If you would normally have a pre-dinner drink at home at 7 p.m., now is the time to have one.

The menu card that you are given after take off will be for 'lunch', but for you it is time for dinner. Plan your meal accordingly and choose those items from the menu that you would normally eat for dinner, as opposed to lunch, and select your wine likewise.

Two to three hours into the flight you will be thinking in terms of 9–10 p.m. Even in summer months, it would now be getting dark at home, so you will wish to minimize light. This is accomplished by picking a port (i.e., left) side seat (looking north as you fly east) so as to avoid the sun. Dinner, followed by reading or a movie, should be taken with the window shade down and the overhead light on. Who knows, you might be surrounded by other jetlag beaters, all with their shades down – thus making it easier for you.

Four to five hours into the flight it is time to start thinking of sleep. You should now take your own combination of nightcap / sleeping pill / herbal hypnotic / melatonin, as described in previous chapters. Go through nightly rituals such as brushing your teeth and using the toilet. You should put your seat in the most horizontal position that you can. If you have an alarm clock on your watch, this should be set to allow you eight hours of sleep. Eyemasks can be deployed to produce darkness. These are often but not invariably essential. Similarly, ear plugs will reduce surrounding noise, thus making it easier to sleep.

This particular flight arrives in Singapore at 0750 hrs, so the plan is to stay asleep as long as possible. You should therefore have previously instructed the cabin crew not to wake you for breakfast. You can have this at Changai airport, or at your hotel on arrival.

An ideal flight from London to Singapore would take off about two hours later, thus allowing you eight hours of sleep, plus time to wake up, have breakfast, and get you in at around 10 a.m. local time.

Meanwhile, the above procedure, planned for BA11, should enable you to be adequately rested and ready to face a full day in Singapore.

Flying west beats jetlag best. This is because, as we saw earlier, flying west elongates your day, and so is less in conflict with your body clock, which is always trying to stretch from the containment of a 24-hour day towards a 25-hour day. Bearing in mind that the same principles would apply to London / San Francisco, and from Paris or Frankfurt or Amsterdam or Madrid or Rome to either San Francisco or Los Angeles, let's conclude by focusing on the following typical long-haul trip westward:

London ✈ Los Angeles

A good flight for this journey would be British Airways BA269, but only if you are a non-smoker. This takes off at 1555 hrs and arrives in Los Angeles at 1855 hrs. If you do smoke, I would suggest Air New Zealand flight NZ1, departing 1720 hrs and arriving 2030 hrs, in preference to British Airways BA283 (departing 1200 and arriving 1500 hrs). This is because it is advisable to catch the latest flight out of London that will still get you in to Los Angeles in time for bed by 11 p.m. local time.

Let's say you don't smoke, and so take BA269. L.A. is eight hours behind London. You therefore stay in bed asleep as long as possible on the morning of your departure. If you get up at 1300 hrs, this is still only 0500 hrs in L.A. Keep everything low-key. Minimum light, and as little noise as possible. Get someone to drive you to the airport, and nap on the way if you can. Take-off time being about 4 p.m. means it is now eight in the morning (for you) and so time to wake up. Accordingly, I would book a port side seat (facing south as you fly west), to benefit from as much sunlight as possible. This is particularly important in winter months when it may already be getting dark at this stage. This is an ideal time to use an artificial light source. Remember that later in the flight you will be willing yourself to stay awake, against your natural inclination, so as much light as possible is helpful.

You must now stay awake during the entire flight.

Eleven hours is a long time, but just think how much work you can get done, and still take in a film or two! I would avoid alcohol on this flight if it tends to make you doze off.

The first meal served tends to be a lunch-type full meal. Turn this as best you can into breakfast by eating the salad, fruit and bread, all with plenty of coffee. Frequent walks up and down the aisle, interacting with your laptop computer, and lively conversations with colleagues or neighbours are just the thing to help you stay awake.

Try to arrange with the cabin staff something approaching a light lunch about six hours into the flight. The last three hours or so of the flight will be gruelling, as your body clock is telling you to shut down and go to sleep. Use every trick in the book to resist this. On touching down in L.A. at about 7 p.m., you have a choice. Ideally you should stay awake until about 11 p.m. local time. This may be quite difficult, as by London time you are really staying up all night. If you succeed in this, do take your melatonin at bedtime, but I don't think you will need anything in the way of pills or alcohol to help you sleep!

Alternatively, at 7 p.m. in L.A., you could decide to crash out immediately. The problem here is to ensure that you don't wake up after eight hours at about four or five in the morning. The answer is to take one of the long-acting sleeping pills, and this should keep you out until about seven or eight o'clock the following morning. Do not take melatonin if you are crashing out at 8 p.m. or you will thoroughly confuse your body clock. Leave the melatonin by your bedside, and if you happen to wake up any time between 11 p.m. and 2 a.m. you can take it then.

The following day, having had at least eight hours sleep one way or the other, things should not be too bad. You will understandably begin to feel tired at about 3 p.m. (11 p.m. London time) so any temptation to nap should be resisted. Thereafter you take melatonin at bedtime for the next three or four nights.

The above examples will hopefully have illustrated how you can put theory into practice. Similar routines, to minimize the effects of jetlag, can be specified for any long-haul flight. Customized recommendations, in accordance with individual needs and personal preferences, can be obtained from the Jetlag Clinic. Please see page 144 for contact details.

15

The Future

Because the importance of the effects of jetlag is being realized by some of those organizations most closely affected by it, a great deal of research has been stimulated in this field, particularly by the air forces of several countries. Understandably, they take a dim view if their fighter pilots crash several millions of pounds worth of aircraft due to error occasioned by jetlag. The perfect chemical cure-all for jetlag is not yet with us, but it may be in the pipeline. Meanwhile, this chapter contains a miscellany of helpful hints and a brief look to the future.

Tyrosine is an amino acid (i.e., one of the building blocks of protein). For some years it has been known that tyrosine protects against the effects of physiological stress.[127] However, more recently it has been established that it can also be used successfully to combat the decline in performance associated with continuing work without sleep.[128] Taken in a dose of approximately 5 grams, the effect has been shown to last for up to three hours.[129] This work has been carried out on U.S. marines training to become pilots. They had been awake for 24 hours continuously by the time the experiment was concluded.

Tyrosine pills are available from health-food shops and do not require a prescription.

Sometimes an overseas business trip will involve a destination at high altitude, such as Mexico City. It is known that travelling to high altitudes reduces the ability to exercise efficiently, and this effect occurs as low as 1500 metres.[130] This has important consequences if your itinerary involves a lot of running around from, say, one plant to another, climbing up and down ladders to inspect machinery. You are more likely to experience physical exhaustion, in addition to the problems of jetlag and sleep deprivation. Help is at hand in the form of humble caffeine. The equivalent of 2–3 cups of percolated coffee has been proved to increase the ability to exercise,[131] but its potential to cause insomnia must be borne in mind when timing its use.

When you arrive at your destination you may, before you go into your first meeting, have a lot of time on your hands. Should you spend this on your own, or mucking in with your travelling companions, or possibly with your hosts?

The evidence is that socializing is an important zeitgeber, such that you are better off (whatever you are doing) in company.[132] Being with other people, particularly strangers, may be the last thing you feel like doing, but if you want to switch your clock more quickly then socializing is strongly recommended.

Unfortunately, many business travellers nowadays will be on medication of one sort or another. It is important that the timing of this medication is not upset by time-zone shifts. Some types of medication will of their very nature need to be adjusted. For example, a traveller who regularly takes a sleeping pill will need to take it at the bedtime of his destination.

Someone taking a blood-pressure medication three time a day will need to take it approximately every eight hours. This will therefore need adjustment when travelling long distances. Remember that when travelling east you shorten your day, and that you lengthen it when travelling west. So if you travel east through eight time zones (e.g., London/Hong Kong) you will need one less dosage in your first day. Equally, when travelling eight time zones west (e.g., London/San Francisco), you will need to take an extra dose in your first day.

Diabetics taking insulin injections will require very careful, precise and individual adjustments of dosage. These are beyond the scope of this book and should be prescribed by the attending physician.

It is very important to maintain physical fitness. Those who exercise regularly to stay fit have higher circadian rhythm amplitudes. Those with a higher rhythm amplitude adapt to shift work more easily and are therefore less subject to jetlag.[133] It is all-too-easy to abandon physical training if you are a frequent flyer. After spending long hours confined in a cabin the last thing you may want is to waste hours in a gym or swimming pool. If so, a long fast walk will do. On arrival at your destination you should take your walk in the afternoon, for an eastward flight, and in the early morning following a westward one.[134]

People with a history of severe depressive or manic-depressive illness should seriously question the wisdom of subjecting themselves to the effects of jetlag on a regular basis. Recurrences of these illnesses are some-times precipitated by travel through a large time-zone difference and more particularly by multiple stop–start flying, as in an around-the-world voyage.[135] It is inter-esting that the direction of travel plays an important part. Travelling east is more likely to precipitate manic changes, while travelling west tends to produces relapses of depression.[136] I have found the flattened mood of minor depressive disorder to be very common amongst patients such as investment bankers who spend a lot of their time in the air. So cheer up! If, while flying west, you *feel* a bit depressed, you probably really are!

Foreign travel frequently involves arriving at a destination that is much hotter or more humid than our home base. Inevitably there will be a large increase in the amount of fluid imbibed. This will usually consist largely of carbonated soft drinks and the question is sometimes raised: do these drinks have a deleterious effect? Apart from the fact that many such drinks contain significant quantities of caffeine (36–48 mgs, compared with 40–108 mgs in a cup of instant coffee or 20–46 mgs in a three-minute-infused cup of tea),[137] they contain an artificial sweetener called aspartame, known commercially as NutraSweet. These drinks have been shown to produce no detectable decline in a variety of intellectual functions.[138]

The race is certainly on to find the ideal jetlag pill. Such a pill should be able to rapidly adjust every function in the body to any given time shift, either backwards or forwards. It should be cheap to manufacture, chemically stable enough to carry around in your pocket all over the world, and it should be free of side effects.

As far back as the 1970s Merck Laboratories were investigating the possible use of a compound called Quiadon.[139] More recently the French company Lafon Laboratories have been testing the possible use of their compound Modafinil.[140]

Such drugs would perform one or other of two functions. Type A drugs would advance or shorten the circadian cycle and so find use in eastbound travel. Drugs found to have this property include the steroid stimulant ACTH,[141] the antidepressant Nomifensine[142] and the anti-asthma drug Theophylline.[143]

Type B drugs, which lengthen the cycle, and could therefore have a use in westward flights, include the anti-mania drug lithium,[144] and the antidepressant Clorgyline.[145] However, before you go running off to your GP asking for handfuls of the above, remember that these developments are still at a very experimental stage and cannot yet be recommended.

Given the resources being allocated to the research, it seems likely that before long a jetlag wonder-drug will be discovered or invented. Meanwhile, it is hoped to update this book on a regular basis, to keep you abreast of new developments in this exciting field.

Appendix A

Sources of Help and Medication

Autohypnosis

The British Society of Medical & Dental Hypnosis can recommend a doctor or dentist in your area who can teach you to hypnotize yourself. You can write to them at (National Office):

17 Keppel ·View Road, Kimberworth, Rotherham, South Yorks, S61 2AR. Tel: 01709–554558.

The Society has a Metropolitan and South Office at:

73 Ware Road, Hertford, Herts, SG13 7ED.

Tel: 0181–905–4342.

Herbal treatments

Details of UK herbalists can be obtained from:

National Institute of Medical Herbalists, 56 Longbrook Street, Exeter, Devon, EX4 6AH. Tel: 01392–426022.

Or from:

The British Herbal Medicine Association, PO Box 304, Bournemouth, Dorset, BH7 6JZ. Tel: 01202–433691.

Light visors, melatonin, self-testing kits

Available from:

The Jetlag Clinic, 41 Elystan Place, Chelsea Green, London, SW3 3JY.

Tel: 0171–584–9779. Fax 0171–584–3779.

For further information on the Jetlag Clinic, please see page 144.

Appendix B: Waking V. Sleeping Strategies

Strategy	For Alertness	For Sleep
Comfort	None	Very comfortable; cosy
Drink	Coffee, chocolate drinks, cola; drinks with caffeine	Alcohol (but not white wine or watery beer)
Drugs	Caffeine, amphetamine	Sleeping pills; antihistamines
Food	Light; sharp tastes; chocolate	Heavy, stodgy food
Gym	Exercise	Massage
Humidity	Dry	Slightly humid
Light	Bright	Dim / dark
Position	Upright	Recumbant
Reading	Work, especially stressful . . .	Soothing novel; poetry
Sound	Talk shows; interactive; rock music	Slow music; Bach, Vivaldi, Mozart
Temperature	Cold	Warm
Washing	Shower, finishing with cold	Hot bath

Appendix C: Sleeping Pills[1]

Drug Name	Speed of Action	Duration of Action (hrs)	Hangover Effect	Side Effects
Bromazepam	Rapid	6–8	None	Unsteadiness
Chloral Hydrate	Very rapid	6–8	None	Stomach upset, flatulence
Chlormethiazole	Rapid	4–6	None	Nasal congestion & itch, conjunctivitis, headache
Chlorpheniramine	Rapid	4–6	Can be marked	Dizziness, impaired reactions
Diphenhydramine	Rapid	4–6	Can be marked	Dizziness, dry mouth
Flunitrazepam	Rapid	8	Very little	Dizziness, headache, unsteadiness
Lormetazepam	Slowish	8–10	Very little	Headache, dizziness
Nitrazepam	Rapid	8–14	Can be marked	Blurred vision, unsteadiness
Oxazepam	Slow	8–10	Little	Unsteadiness, dizziness
Promethazine	Rapid	4–6	Can be marked	Dizziness, dry mouth
Temazepam	Rapid	8–10	Very little	Unsteadiness, dizziness
Zolpidem	Rapid	3–6	None	Stomach upset, dizziness, headache
Zopiclone	Rapid	4–7	None	Metallic aftertaste, nausea, headache

[1] Sources: Goodman & Gilman, The Pharmacological Basis of Therapeutics, McGraw-Hill, 9th edition, 1996; Laurence & Bennett, Clinical Pharmacology, Churchill Livingstone, 1996; Association of the British Pharmaceutical Industry, Compendium of Data Sheets, 1996–7, Datapharm Publications Ltd, London.

Appendix D

Autoimmune Diseases

In Chapter 9 it was suggested that, in the present state of knowledge, patients suffering from any autoimmune disease should not take supplementary melatonin. Some of the more common autoimmune diseases are:

Chronic active hepatitis
Dermatomyositis
Hashimoto's thyroditis
Multiple sclerosis
Myasthenia gravis
Pernicious anaemia
Polyarteritis nodosa
Primary bilary cirrhosis
Rheumatoid arthritis
Scleroderma
Sjogren's syndrome
Systemic lupus erythematosis

There are a number of rarer autoimmune diseases, and it is possible that others may be identified in the future. If you know you have a medical condition, check with your doctor that it is not an autoimmune disease before you take supplementary melatonin.

References

Chapter 1: The Normal Circadian Rhythm

1. Horne, J.A., et al, 'A self-assessment questionnaire to determine morningness-eveningness in human circadian rhythms', *International Journal of Chronobiology* 1976 (4), pp.97–110.

2. Horne, J.A., et al, 'Individual differences in human circadian rhythms', *Biological Psychiatry*, 1977 (5), pp.179–90.

3. Monk, T.H., 'Shift Work', in *Principles and Practice of Sleep Medicine*, W.B. Saunders & Co., 1989, pp.332–7.

4. Manchester, W., *The Caged Lion: Winston Spencer Churchill 1932–1940*, Cardinal Books, 1988.

5. Personal communication to the author.

6. Cosgrove, P., *Margaret Thatcher, A Tory and Her Party*, Hutchinson & Co., London, 1978, p.22.

7. Kleitman, N., *Sleep and Wakefulness*, University of Chicago Press, Illinois, 1939.

8. Berkson, J., et al, 'Intra-daily variability of basal metabolism', *American Journal of Physiology*, 1938 (121), p.669.

9. Kleitman, N., et al, 'The establishment of the diurnal temperature cycle', *American Journal of Physiology*, 1937 (199), p.48.

10. Kleitman, N., et al, *Sleep Characteristics*, University of Chicago Press, 1934.

11. Regelsberger, *Ergebnisse de Internal Medicine*, 1935 (48), p.125.

12. Luckhardt, A., et al, 'Studies in gastric secretion', *American Journal of Physiology*, 1924 (70), p.174.

13. Strughold, H., 'Physiological day-night cycle in global flights', *Aviation Medicine*, 1952 (October), p.464.

14. Forsgren, E., 'Rhythmicity of liver function and of internal metabolism', *Archives Medicine Scandinavica*, 1934 (29), p.95.

15. Aschoff, J., 'Circadian rhythms in man', *Science*, 1965 (148), pp.1427–32.

16. Wever R., *The Circadian System of Man: Results of experiments under temporal isolation*, Springer Verlag, New York, 1979.

Chapter 2: The Flying Revolution

17. Runes, D.D., *The Diary and Sundry Observations of Thomas Alva Edison*, New York Philosophical Library, 1948.

Chapter 3: Jetlag Vulnerability & Symptoms

18. Graeber, R.C., et al, *Alterations in performance following rapid transmeridian flight. Rhythmic aspects of behaviour.* Erbaum Associates, 1982, pp.173–212.

19. Holley, D.C., et al, 'Effects of circadian rhythms phase alteration on physiological and psychological variables', NASA Technical Memorandum TN–81277, 1981.

20. Raboutet, J., et al, 'Trouble du sommeil et du rhythme de vie chez le personnel navigant effectuant de vol à longue distance', *Medical Aeronautica*, 1985 (13), pp.311–22.

21. Gander, H., et al, 'Age, circadian rhythms and sleep loss in flight crews', *Aviation Space and Environmental Medicine*, 1993 (64), pp.189–95.

22. Wright, J.E., et al, 'Effect of travel across time zones on exercise capacity and performance', *Aviation Space and Environmental Medicine*, 1983 (54), pp.132–7.

23. Haugli, L., et al, 'Health sleep and mood perceptions reported by airline crews flying short and long hauls', *Aviation Space and Environmental Medicine*, 1994 (65), pp.27–34.

24. Dyregrov, A., et al, 'Fear of flying in civil aviation personnel', *Aviation Space and Environmental Medicine*, 1992 (63), pp.831–8.

25. Preston, F.S., 'Temporal Discord', *Journal of Psychosomatic Research*, 1978 (22), pp.377–83.

26. Hauty, G.T., et al, 'Phase shifts of the human circadian system and performance deficit during the periods of transition', *Aerospace Medicine*, 1966 (73), pp.1257–62.

27. Graeber, R.C., et al, *Human Eating Behaviour*, Food Sciences Laboratory, 1978. Technical Report Natick/TR–78/o22.

28. Haugli, L., et al, *op. cit.*

29. Preston, F.S., et al, 'Effects of flying and of time changes on menstrual length and performance in airline stewardesses', *Aerospace Medicine*, 1973 (44), pp.438–43.

30. Shmidova, V.F., 'The effect of high altitude and high speed flights on the functioning of air hostesses' obstetric organs', *Gig Truda Professional Zabologue*, 1966 (10), pp.55–7.

31. Beljan, J.R., et al, *Human Performance in the Aviation Environment*, NASA, NAS2–6657, 1972.

32. Elliot, A., et al, 'Effects of real and simulated time zone shifts upon circadian rhythms of body temperature, plasma 11-hydroxycorticosteroids and renal excretion in human subjects', *Journal of Physiology*, 1972 (221), pp.227–57.

33. Stepanova, S.I., 'Effect of transmeridian flight on the human body', *Kosmologica Biologica Aviaksom Medicine*, 1974 (8), pp.3–12.

34. Klein, K.E., et al, 'Circadian rhythms of pilots' efficiency and effects of multiple time-zone travel', *Aerospace Medicine*, 1970 (41), pp.125–32.

35. Klein, K.E., et al, 'Significance of circadian rhythms in aerospace operations', AGARDograph No.247, Advisory Group for Aerospace Research and Development, NATO, 1980.

36. Stepanova, S.I., *Problems of Space Biology*, Moscow Izdatelstvo Nauka, 1977.

37. Andlauer, P., et al, 'Amplitude of the oral temperature, circadian rhythm and tolerance of shiftwork', *Chronobiologia*, 1979 (6, supplement 1), p.67–73.

38. Hauty, G.T., et al, 'Phase shifts of the human circadian system and performance deficit during the periods of transition', *Aerospace Medicine*, 1966 (73), pp.1257–62.

39. Folkhard, S., et al, 'Towards a predictive test of adjustment to shift work', *Ergonomics*, 1979 (22), pp.79–91.

40. Colquhoun, W.P., 'Phase shift in temperature rhythm after transmeridian flight, as related to pre-flight phase angle', *International Archives of Occupational and Environmental Health*, 1979 (42), pp.149–57.

41. Colquhoun, W.P., 'Rhythms in Performance', in *Biological Rhythms*, Plenum Press, New York, 1981, Vol.4, pp.333–48.

42. Winget, C.M., et al, 'Influence of 105 days of social deprivation on physiological rhythmicity', *Aerospace Medical Association Preprints*, 1974, pp.87–8.

43. Knutsson, A., et al, 'Increased risk of ischemic heart disease in shift workers', *Lancet*, 1986, pp.89–92.

44. Taylor, P.J., et al, 'Mortality of shift and day workers 1956–1968', *British Journal of Industrial Medicine*, 1972 (29), pp.1441–3.

45. Band, P.R., et al, 'Cohort study of Air Canada pilots; mortality, cancer incidence and leukemia risk', *American Journal of Epidemiology*, 1996, (143 no.2), pp.137–43.

Chapter 4: Some Statistics

46. *World Air Transport Statistics*, International Air Transport Association, 1996, No.40.

47. *Annual Statement of Movements, Passengers and Cargo 1994*, Civil Aviation Authority, London, 1995.

48. *Daily Telegraph*, London, 23 April 1996.

49. Conroy, R.T., 'Time zone transitions and business executives', *Transactions of the Society of Occupational Medicine*, 1971 (21), pp.69–72.

50. Reuters News, Washington, February 1992.

51. Reuters News, Moscow, January 1992.

52. *Time*, 26 April 1982.

53. *Financial Times*, London, 26 & 27 November 1994.

Chapter 5: Adverse Effects of Flying

54. Johnson, R., et al, *Travel Fitness*, Human Kinetics, Champaign Illinois, 1995, p.20.

55. McFarland, R.A., 'Influence of changing time zones on air crew and passengers', *Aerospace Medicine*, 1974 (45 no.6), pp.648–58.

56. McFarland, R.A., 'The effects of altitude on pilots' performance', *Aviation and Space Medicine*, Oslo Universitetsforlaget, 1969, pp.96–108.

57. Denison, D.M., et al, 'Complex reaction times at simulated cabin altitudes of 5000 ft and 8000 ft', *Aerospace Medicine*, 1966 (37), pp.1010–13.

58. Best, A.S., 'Pan American World Airways air-conditioning tests during revenue flights', *Aviation Space and Environmental Medicine*, 1980 (2), p.170.

59. Xenex Corporation, *Aircraft-Specific Climate Factors*, Aviation Safety and Health Association, 1989 (1), p.2.

60. McFarland, R.A., et al, 'Alterations in dark adaptation under reduced oxygen tensions', *American Journal of Physiology*, 1939 (127), pp.37–50.

61. *Airliner Cabin Environment, Air Quality and Safety*, Board on Environmental Studies and Toxicology, National Research Counsel, Washington D.C., 1986, p.119.

62. Mar, J., 'Risk of acquiring respiratory tract infections during air travel', *Journal of the American Medical Association*, 1987 (258), p.2764.

63. Davies, I.D., et al, 'The mortality of British Airways pilots, 1966–1989; a proportional mortality study', *Aviation Space and Environmental Medicine*, 1992 (63), p.276–9.

64. James, P.B., 'Jet lag, pulmonary embolism and hypoxia', *Lancet*, 1996 (347), p.1697.

65. Band, P.R., et al, *op. cit.*.

Chapter 6: The Strategies

66. Nicholson, A.N., et al, 'Sleep after transmeridian flights', *Lancet*, 22 November 1986, pp.1205–8.

67. Desir, D., et al, 'Effects of jetlag on hormonal patterns', *Journal of Clinical and Endocrinological Metabolism*, 1981 (52), p.628–41.

Chapter 8: To Sleep, To Wake

68. Montileone, P., et al, 'Physical exercise at night blunts the nocturnal increase of plasma melatonin levels in healthy humans', *Life Sciences*, 1990 (47), pp.1989–95.

69. Van Cauter, E., 'Phase shifting of light and exercise on the human circadian clock', Chicago University Department of Medicine, 1992. Annual report no. AFOSR–TR 92–1665.

70. Coren, S., *Sleep Thieves*, Free Press, 1996, p.162.

71. Komblueh, I.H., et al, 'Artificial air ionization in physical medicine', *American Journal of Physical Medicine*, 1955 (34), pp.618–24.

72. Hildebrandt, G., et al, 'Twelve and twenty-four hour rhythms in error frequency of locomotive drivers and the influence of tiredness', *International Journal of Chronobiology*, 1974 (2), pp.175–80.

73. Coren, S., *op. cit.*, p.159.

74. Ehret, C.F., et al, 'Consideration of diet in alleviating jetlag', in *Principles and Applications to Shifts in Schedules*, Sijthoff and Noordhooff, 1980, pp.393–402.

75. Emonson, D.L., et al, 'The use of amphetamines in the U.S. Air Force tactical operations during Desert Shield and Storm', *Aviation Space and Environmental Medicine*, 1995 (66), pp.260–3.

76. Laurence, D.R., *Clinical Pharmacology*, Churchill Livingstone, 1996.

Chapter 9: Melatonin

77. Waldhauser, F., et al, 'Sleep laboratory investigations on hypnotic properties of melatonin', *Psychopharmacology*, 1990 (100), pp.222–6.

78. Dahlitz, M., 'Delayed sleep phase syndrome response to melatonin', *Lancet*, 1991 (337), pp.1121–4.

79. Garfinkel, D., et al, 'Improvement of sleep quality in elderly people by controlled-release melatonin', *Lancet*, 1995 (346), pp.541–3.

80. Arendt, J., et al, 'Some effects of jetlag and their alleviation by melatonin', *Ergonomics*, 1987 (30), pp.1379–93.

81. Petrie, K., et al, 'Effect of melatonin on jetlag after long-haul flights', *British Medical Journal*, 1989 (298), pp.705–7.

82. Lieberman, H.R, et al, 'Effects of melatonin on human mood and performance', *Brain Research*, 1984 (323), pp.201–7.

83. Barchas, J., et al, 'Acute pharmacology of melatonin', *Nature*, 1967 (214), pp.919–20.

84. Waldhauser, F., *The Pineal Gland*, Raven Press, New York, 1984, pp.345–69.

85. Constantinescu, C.S., 'Melanin, melatonin, MSH and the susceptibility to autoimmune demylenination', *Medical Hypotheses*, 1995 (45), pp.455–8.

86. Hansson, I., et al, 'The pineal hormone melatonin exaggerates development of collagen-induced arthritis in mice', *Journal of Immunology*, 1992 (39), pp.23–30.

87. Arendt, J., et al, 'Alleviation of jetlag by melatonin; preliminary results of controlled double-blind trail', *British Medical Journal*, 1986 (292), p.1170.

88. Petrie, K., et al, *op. cit.*

89. Lino, A., et al, 'Melatonin and jetlag: treatment schedule', *Biological Psychiatry*, 1993 (34), pp.587–8.

90. Claustrat, B., et al, 'Melatonin and jetlag: confirmatory result using a simplified protocol', *Biological Psychiatry*, 1992 (32), pp.705–11.

91. Aldous, M., et al, 'Plasma concentrations of melatonin in man following oral absorption of different preparations', *British Journal of Clinical Pharmacology*, 1985 (19), pp.517–21.

92. MacFarlane, J.G., et al, 'The effects of exogenous melatonin on the total sleep time and daytime alertness of chronic insomniacs: a preliminary study', *Biological Psychiatry*, 1991 (30), pp.371–6.

93. Short, R,V., 'Melatonin: hormone of darkness', *British Medical Journal*, 1993 (307), pp.952–3.

Chapter 10: Light

94. Lewy, A.J., et al, 'Light suppresses melatonin secretion in humans', *Science*, 1980 (210), pp.1267–9.

95. Lemmar, B., et al, 'Effects of bright light on circadian patterns of cyclic adenosine monophosphate, melatonin and cortisol in healthy subjects', *European Journal of Endocrinology*, 1994 (130 no.5), pp.472–7.

96. Bojkowski, C.J., et al, 'Suppression of nocturnal plasma melatonin and 6-sulphatoxymelatonin by bright light and dim light in man', *Hormone and Metabolic Research*, 1987 (19), pp.437–40.

97. Czeisler, C., et al, 'Bright light induction of strong (type 0) resetting of the human circadian pacemaker', *Science*, 1989 (244), pp.1328–33.

Chapter 11: Sleep Deprivation

98. Carskadon, M.A., et al, 'Cumulative effects of sleep restriction on daytime sleepiness', *Psychophysiology* 1981 (18 no.2), pp.107–11.

99. Dinges, D.F., et al, 'Performing while sleepy; effects of experimentally induced sleepiness', in *Sleep, Sleepiness and Performance*, John Wiley & Sons Ltd, Chichester, 1991, pp.97–128.

100. Tilley, A., et al, 'Sleep Deprivation' in *Handbook of Human Performance*, Academic Press, 1992, pp.237–59.

101. Moore-Ede, M., *The 24 Hour Society*, Piatkus, 1993.

Chapter 12: Women & Jetlag

102. Caplan, G., 'Psychological aspects of pregnancy', in *The Psychological Basis of Medical Practice*, Harper and Row, New York, pp.441–7.

103. Young, D.M., 'Psychiatric morbidity in travelers to Honolulu Hawaii', *Comprehensive Psychiatry*, 1995 (36 no.3), pp.224–8.

104. Dennis, J., 'The physiology and management of the puerperium', in *Obstetrics* by Turnbull and Chamberlain, Churchill Livingstone, 1989, p.899.

105. Cameron, R.G., 'Should air hostesses continue flight duty during the first trimester of pregnancy?', *Aerospace Medicine*, 1973 (44 no.5), pp.552–6.

106. Laurence, D.L., *Clinical Pharmacology*, Churchill Livingstone, 1992, p.346.

107. Lewis, P.G., 'Adverse effects of drugs on the foetus', in *Clinical Pharmacology in Obstetrics*, Wright, PSG, 1983, p.17.

108. Compendium of Data Sheets, Association of the British Pharmaceutical Industry, Datapharm, 1997, p.309.

109. Ibid., pp.551–2.

110. Ibid., pp.882–3.

111. Ibid., p.882.

112. Ibid., pp.871–2.

113. Ibid., pp.851–2.

114. *Drugs and Therapeutics Bulletin*, 1996 (34 no.4), pp.30–2

115. Preston, F.S., 'Effects of flying and of time changes on the menstrual cycle length and performance in airline stewardesses', *Aerospace Medicine*, 1973 (44), pp.438–43.

116. Shmidova, V.F., *op. cit.*

117. Haugli, L., et al, *op. cit.*

118. Guillebaud, J., *Contraception · Your Questions Answered*, Churchill Livingstone, 1994, p.245.

119. Cruickshank, J.M., et al, 'Air travel and thrombotic episodes, the economy class syndrome', *Lancet*, 1988 (2), pp.497–8.

120. Eddy, J., *Obstetrics and Gynaecology in General Practice*, Churchill Livingstone, 1987, pp.261–2.

121. Walsh, P.C., et al, *Campbell's Urology*, W.B. Saunders & Co., 1994, pp.2091–2.

Chapter 13: Alcohol

122. Kozararevic, D., et al, 'Frequency of alcohol consumption and morbidity and mortality', *Lancet*, 1980 (1), pp.613–6.

123. Klatsky, A.L., et al, 'Alcohol and mortality', *Annals of Internal Medicine*, 1992 (117), pp.646–54.

124. Yesavage, J., et al, 'Hangover effects on aircraft pilots 14 hours after alcohol ingestion', *American Journal of Psychology*, 1986 (143), pp.1546–50.

125. Goldberg, D., et al, *Psychiatry in Medical Practice*, Routledge, 1994, pp.188–9.

126. Young, D.M., *op. cit.*.

Chapter 15: The Future

127. Banderet, L.E., et al, 'Treatment with tyrosine, a neurotransmitter precursor, reduces environmental stress in humans', *Brain Research Bulletin*, 1989 (22), pp.759–62.

128. Owasoyo, J.O., et al, 'Tyrosine and its potential use as a countermeasure to performance decrement in military sustained operations', *Aviation Space and Environmental Medicine*, 1992 (63), pp.364–9.

129. Neri, D.F., et al, 'The effects of tyrosine on cognitive performance during extended wakefulness', *Aviation Space and Environmental Medicine*, 1995 (April), pp.313–9.

130. Young, A.J., et al, 'Human acclimatization to high terrestrial altitude', in *Human Performance, Physiology and Environmental*

Medicine at Terrestrial Extremes, Benchmark Press, Indianapolis, 1988, pp.497–543.

131. Fulco, C.S., et al, 'Effect of caffeine on submaximal exercise performance at altitude', *Aviation Space and Environmental Medicine*, 1994 (June), pp.539–45.

132. Wever, R., *The Circadian System of Man; Results of Experiments under Temporal Isolation*, Springer Verlag, New York, 1979.

133. Atkinson, G., et al, 'A comparison of circadian rhythms in work performance between physically active and inactive subjects', *Ergonomics*, 1993 (36), pp.273–81.

134. Ferrer, C.F., et al, 'Circadian-rhythm desynchronosis in military deployments: a review of current strategies', *Aviation Space and Environmental Medicine*, 1995 (66 no.6), pp571–8.

135. Monden M.A., et al, 'Mental decompensation during vacation abroad', *Nederlands Tijdschrift voor Geneeskunde*, 1994 (July) pp.1520–3.

136. Young, D.M., *op. cit.*.

137. Food Technologists Expert Panel 1987. Consumer Reports 1991.

138. Stokes, A.F., et al, 'Effects of acute aspartame and acute alcohol ingestion upon the cognitive performance of pilots', *Aviation Space and Environmental Medicine*, 1991 (July) pp.648–53.

139. Simpson, H.W., et al, 'Double-blind trial of a possible chronobiotic, Quiadon', Field studies in N. W. Greenland, *International Journal of Chronobiology*, 1973 (1), pp.287–311.

140. Lyons, T.J., et al, 'Modafinil; the unique properties of a new stimulant', *Aviation Space and Environmental Medicine*, 1991 (May), pp.432–5.

141. Andrews, R.V., 'Temporal secretory responses of cultured hamster adrenals', *Comparative Biochemistry and Physiology*, 1968 (26), pp.179–93.

142. Halberg, F., et al, 'Glossary of chronobiology', *Chronobiology*, 1977 (4, supplement 1), pp.1–189.

143. Ehret, C.F., et al, 'Chronotypic action of Theophyline and of Pentobarbitol as circadian zeitgebers in the rat', *Science*, 1975 (188), pp.1212–14.

144. Kripke, D.F., et al, 'Lithium slows rat circadian activity', *Life Sciences*, 1980 (27), pp.1319–21.

145. Wirz-Justice, A., et al, 'Antidepressant drugs can slow or dissociate circadian rhythms', *Experientia*, 1982 (38), pp.1301–9.

Readers' Notes

The two blank pages following are provided for you to note any personally useful information such as flight details, sleeping v. waking schedules, meeting times, and so forth.

THE JETLAG CLINIC

Founded by Dr O'Connell in 1996, the Jetlag Clinic specializes in providing planning and treatment for passengers undertaking international flights. All medications are provided on-site, and protocols are constantly updated as new research indicates more efficacious methods for eliminating jetlag.

Treatments are administered and flight plans are devised in accordance with each traveller's unique requirements and medical history. Inquiries are welcome from private individuals and also from companies on behalf of their directors and employees.

Contact:

   The Jetlag Clinic
   41 Elystan Place
   Chelsea Green
   London
   SW3 3JY

   Tel: 0171–584–9779. Fax 0171–584–3779.

EMAIL ADDRESS:

david.oconnell@dial.pipex.com

Or for the latest updates on medications, treatments and information services available, visit our web site at:

http://dspace.dial.pipex.com/david.oconnell